The Least Likely Man

Marshall Nirenberg and the Discovery of the Genetic Code

Franklin H. Portugal

The MIT Press
Cambridge, Massachusetts
London, England

MIT Press books may be purchased at special quantity discounts for business or sales promotional use. For information, please email special_sales@mitpress.mit.edu.

This book was set in Stone by the MIT Press. Printed and bound in the United States of America.

Library of Congress Cataloging-in-Publication Data

Portugal, Franklin H., author.
The least likely man : Marshall Nirenberg and the discovery of the genetic code / Franklin H. Portugal.
    pages   cm
Includes bibliographical references and index.
ISBN 978-0-262-02847-9 (hardcover : alk. paper)
1. Nirenberg, Marshall W. 2. Biochemists—United States—Biography.
3. Geneticists—United States—Biography. 4. Genetic code. I. Title.
QP511.8.N57P67   2015
576.5092—dc23
[B]
2014017232
10 9 8 7 6 5 4 3 2 1

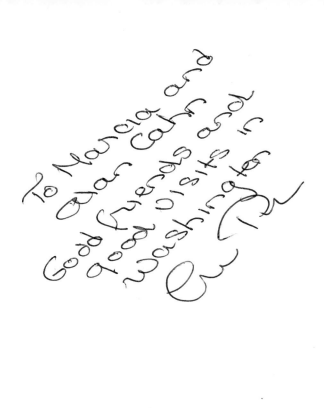

To Marcia and
Brian Cahn
Good Friends and
good visits in
Washington

The Least Likely Man

In loving memory of my parents, Henrietta and Morris Portugal, and Sylvia and Sol Howard, who gave me Evelyn

Contents

Acknowledgments

In the three years it took to write this book, many people contributed their professional skills and/or reminiscences to make it all possible. I acknowledge with pleasure each and every one.

Family

Ana Bonnheim, Bonnie Bonheim, Malcolm Bonnheim, Noah Bonnheim, Joan Geiger, and Myrna Weissman.

Interviews

Bernard Agranoff, Bruce Ames, Samuel Barondes, Arthur Beaudet, Stanley Becker, Alvin Blocker, Rodney Blocker, James Boyles, Thomas Caskey, Brian Clark, Minor Judd Coon, David Davies, Gary Felsenfeld, Robert Gallo, Joseph Goldstein, Linda Greenhouse, Dolph Hatfield, Arthur Hillman, William Jakoby, Oliver Jones, Edward Kravitz, Karl Krueger, Philip Leder, Judith Levin, Richard Marshall, Robert Martin, Heinrich Matthaei, Matthew Meselson, Charles O'Neal, Phillip Nelson, Alan Peterkofsky, Fritz Rottman, Alessandra Rovescalli, Edward Scolnick, Melvin Shader, Millicent Tomkins, Joel Trupin, Conrad Wagner, Arthur Weissbach, Herbert Weissbach, and Bernard Witkop.

James Watson and Sydney Brenner—the two living members of the RNA Tie Club—were contacted for an interview for this book on a number of occasions. Unfortunately, James Watson was unavailable, and Sydney Brenner did not respond to my requests.

Libraries and Archives

Phyllis Andrews, University of Rochester; Frank Ascione, University of Michigan; Marcia Bassett, Barnard College; Jim Berry, Roger Tory Peterson

Institute; Chip Calhoun, American Institute of Physics; Cynthia Cardona-Meléndez, Orange County Regional History Center; John Carter, Columbia University; H. Frederick Dylla, American Institute of Physics; Jean Ferguson, Duke University Archives; Stephanie Gaub, Orange County Regional History Center; James Gehrlich, New York-Presbyterian/Weill Cornell; Gianna Gifford, Boston Public Library; Ana Guimaraes, Cornell University; Dane Guerrero, Hunter College; Victoria A. Harden, Office of NIH History and Stetten Museum; Barbara Faye Harkins, Office of NIH History; Alice Harmon, University of Florida; Julio L. Hernandez-Delgado, Hunter College; Karen L. Jania, University of Michigan; Garret B. Kremer-Wright, Orange County Regional History Center; Peggy McBride, University of Florida; Amy McDonald, Duke University Archives; Sharon C. Mathis, Office of NIH History and Stetten Museum; Nicole Milano, New York University; Christie Moffat, National Library of Medicine; Malgosia Myc, University of Michigan; Brian McNerny, Lydon Baines Johnson Library; Mary Frances O'Brien, Boston Public Library; Mark Palmer, Alabama Department of Archives and History; Ludmila Pollock, Cold Spring Harbor Laboratory; Tana M. Porter, Orange County Regional History Center; John Rees, National Library of Medicine; Emily Sanford, U. of Michigan; Crystal Smith, National Library of Medicine; Adam J. Stone, City College of New York; Paul Theerman, National Library of Medicine; Linda Todd, The Catholic University of America; Sara Van Arsdel, Orange County Regional History Center; Debra Wilkins, Alabama Department of Archives and History; and John Zarrillo, Cold Spring Harbor Laboratory.

MIT Press

Christopher Eyer, Robert Prior, and Marcy Ross.

Museums

Normal I. Platnick, American Museum of Natural History; Ward Wheeler, American Museum of Natural History; and Marcia Jo Zerivitz, Jewish Museum of Florida.

Research and Transcription

Julius Adler, Falvia J. Arana, Laurence Auerbach, Edwin Becker, Margaret Boehm, Arielle Capurso, Sean Carroll, Christopher Cleary, Francis Collins, Mathew Daniels, Christopher Donohue, Matthew Dugandzic, Vicky

Guo, Norma Zabriskie Heaton, Haruhiro Higashida, Kenneth Kreuzer, Peter Lengyel, Howard Markel, Judy Mermelstein, Jennifer Murduck, Toshiharu Nagatsu, Frank Nordllie, Joseph Perpich, Carlos Basilio Reyes, Alexander Rich, Steven Sabol, Alan Schechter, Shail K. Sharma, Phillip A. Sharp, William L. Smith, Vassiliki Betty Smocovitis, Harold Varmus, and Victor Vogel.

Thanks Go as Well to the Individuals Below

Yale Altman, Katherine D. Anderson, Robert Balaban, Otis Brawley, Cindy Cissel, Jack Cohen, Irwin Feldman, Hank Grasso, Bruce Howard, Evelyn Howard, Orest Hurko, Michael Kancher, Ian Lowe, Joseph E. Nascimento, Laura Patricio, Herman S. Paul, Daniel P. Scott, Mini Shader, Walter Reich, Victor Vogel, Marc-Denis Weitze, Morgan Woerner, and Phil Wolgel.

Any omission is inadvertent and very much regretted.

Introduction

Marshall Warren Nirenberg is the most famous person you have never heard of. In 1968, he shared the Nobel Prize for discovery of the alphabet of life—the genetic code. That discovery has had an almost immeasurable impact, not just in science, but on society as a whole. It is the Rosetta Stone on which we interpret the 3.3 billion letters of DNA, the genetic material that makes us human.

Then why is Marshall so little known? In this book, that is one of several questions I have sought to answer.

And who really discovered the genetic code? That is an equally important question. Despite awarding the Nobel Prize to Marshall Nirenberg and others, that question continues to prove contentious. Matt Ridley, supported by the Alfred P. Sloan Foundation in New York, claims Francis Crick was first.[1] Crick was also the co-discoverer of the spiral staircase structure of DNA and a Nobel Laureate. Sydney Brenner, another Nobel Laureate, has also laid claim to the genetic code.[2] Who is right?

If Marshall was first, how and when did he do it? What makes the man who makes the ideas? Where did his ideas come from? When and how did they develop? How did he nurture them? What caused them to shrivel at times? How did they survive the stifling winds of competition? How, indeed, did he ever triumph?

No one in his entire life ever voted Marshall "most likely to succeed." If he was understated, he was also constantly underrated. He was modest, perhaps to a fault. But he was also clever and creative. Marshall did something prescient, something somewhat unusual for a scientist. In addition to his lab notebooks, he kept a separate set of green, hardcover notebooks. Into those notebooks tumbled a steady stream of ideas, thoughts, and concerns. A careful reading of those entries has supplied much of the material on which this book is based. I have used that material to try to provide answers to the questions I have posed.

Rather than a broad view of science, I have used Marshall Nirenberg's story to illustrate how science gets done. This book is certainly not the first attempt to do so. But perhaps it takes a bit of a different tack. I have sought to provide a critical analysis of the various claims and counterclaims based on my own background as a scientist. Rather than simply depending on the reminiscences of men years after the fact regarding who was first to make each discovery, I have gone back to original source materials. What did they say and do at the time, not just what did they remember afterwards? I have included the good, the bad, and the ugly.

Perhaps I hold a slight advantage for telling Marshall's story. I was a participant in his lab at a critical time: one year before he won the Nobel Prize and another year after. I thus had a ringside seat not only to Marshall's work on the genetic code but on his immediate transition to a whole new field of biology, the study of how the brain functions. Over the next 40 years, I periodically stayed in touch with him. Finally, I had one last conversation with Marshall five days before he died.

A lot of drama is tucked into Marshall's story. An almost deathly chill as a child. A swamp rat as a teenager. On the cusp of solving one of the most difficult and significant problems of 20th-century biology while barely out of graduate school. And opposed by no less than seven Nobel Laureates. Then, a Nobel Laureate himself. Now almost forgotten.

Despite my long association with Marshall Nirenberg, I hope to have written a balanced account. I have tried to be just as critical yet fair about him as I have with others in his story. My hope is that I have succeeded. My fear is that I may not have. I leave it to the reader to draw his or her own conclusions.

1   A New Age

In 1927, the year of Marshall Warren Nirenberg's birth, New York City welcomed in the New Year in "a misty, insidiously soaking rain." Hotels reported a record attendance for the celebration. Nightclubs enjoyed solid bookings despite their soaring prices, theaters recorded one of their best nights ever, and movies worked overtime with midnight shows added. The city had to add 1,000 extra traffic men to handle the heavy stream of cars and the traffic snarls.[1]

Despite warnings of poisoned liquor—for Prohibition enacted through the Eighteenth Amendment to the US Constitution almost a decade earlier still held sway—New Yorkers indulged freely at private parties and the numerous speakeasies. Bellevue Hospital braced to handle cases of overindulgence and those caused by bad liquor.[1]

The passage of this New Year's Eve caused another celebration. A radio message sent during a New Year's celebration from a ship anchored in New Zealand flew halfway around the world to the Associated Press in New York. However, because of the time difference, the message arrived hours before the New Year's celebration in New York had begun. The feat, said David Sarnoff, general manager of the Radio Corporation of America, provided proof-of-principle by which short-wave communication held the promise to greatly enable news-gathering around the world.[2]

Into this world, and into the city of New York, Marshall arrived on April 10, 1927. His birth took place at the New York Nursery and Child's Hospital at Lexington Avenue and 51st Street.[3] Marshall's birth certificate indicated that the family lived at 812 East 22nd Street in Brooklyn. Marshall's father, Harry Nirenberg, was 30 years old; his mother, Minerva Nirenberg, just 22. She listed her occupation as housewife.

A little more than a month after Marshall's birth, on May 21, 1927, the aviator Charles Lindbergh landed his Spirit of St. Louis near Paris, completing the first solo airplane flight across the Atlantic Ocean.[4] When he landed in Paris, a crowd of 100,000 people gathered at Le Bourget Airfield and charged toward his plane in what the *New York Times* called a "movement of humanity."

In terms of health statistics, it seemed to be a good time to be born. In 1927, New York City reported the lowest death rate in its history for infants less than one year old. Of every 1,000 children in this age group, only 56 died. The death rate among children ages one to five years was also the lowest ever recorded in the city. The reduction, said Health Commissioner Louis Harris, could be attributed to parents who "today are more insistent than ever in providing adequately for their offspring."[5]

And not just for children did the expectations of world health brighten. In Paris, Professor Teissier praised recent advances leading rapidly to the extinction of epidemics. This was, he said, the result of colonial sanitation and the work of doctors in the World War. Though smallpox was almost negligible during the war, typhoid fever had been checked by inoculations. Influenza, he noted, was the signal exception "escaping the bonds of science."[6]

Meanwhile, it was the exciting, high-flying "Roaring Twenties" in America and Europe. The years after World War I brought dramatic changes. After decades of struggle, women finally received the vote. American households changed too, embracing a surge in consumer products that brought automobiles, telephones, and modern kitchen appliances to many homes for the first time. A culture of celebrity arose as well. Sports figures like Babe Ruth and Jack Dempsey became household names, and film actors were media darlings who filled grand movie palaces.

Marshall's Family History

Even in 1927, the complete genealogy of Marshall's family seemed complicated and somewhat obscure. The one overriding theme to the clan's evolution appeared to be immigration from Eastern Europe to America. This came about more as a push out of their native countries rife with anti-Semitism than as a pull toward the opportunities found in this country. The family believed the Nirenberg clan dated back to Mordechai who owned a hotel in Brest, which stood on the Russian-Polish border. In 1802, a fire destroyed a large part of the Jewish quarter. About two decades later, fire again destroyed a great number of the Jewish buildings of Brest, among them five houses of prayer.[7]

Yet, the Jews of Brest were indefatigable. They built a Jewish Hospital, with 40 beds, and a pharmacy, supported by income from the meat tax and from voluntary contributions. Thirteen years later, a new synagogue arose, followed in succeeding decades by an asylum for widows, dispensary, poorhouse, and a Jewish school for 500 pupils. A half century later, voluntary contributions still managed to maintain all these institutions.[7]

Marshall's great-grandfather on his father's side of the family, Abraham Nirenberg, owned a store 15 miles from Odessa, a major seaport on the Black Sea in the Ukraine. The presence of the first Jews in Odessa dated back to 1789. By the outbreak of World War II, Jews made up 30 percent of Odessa's population.[8] From the start, the Jews from Odessa engaged in export and wholesale trade, banking and industry, the liberal professions and crafts. But life there could be tenuous. Anti-Jewish outbreaks occurred periodically in Odessa, as well as many other attempted attacks or unsuccessful efforts to provoke them.[8]

Abraham married Anna, and they had three children: Max, Lou, and Nathan. At age 16, Max emigrated by himself from Odessa because of the latest pogrom (organized massacres of Jews) and possibly to avoid being drafted into the Russian army. He arrived in Philadelphia in 1888, and then went to New York. There, he secured a job sweeping floors in a shirt factory. With time, Max rose through the company ranks and did so well that he eventually bought the factory and established Lion Brand Shirts, a nationally distributed line. In the 1950s, he sold his company to a top national shirt manufacturer.

Max married Fannie Cisin who had immigrated from Starokonstantinov, Russia, near Odessa. Max and Fannie eventually had six children, Arthur, Harry, Bert, Frank, Dave, and Clara. Harry would become Marshall's father.

In 1920, the Nirenbergs lived on Newkirk Avenue in Brooklyn. The family must have prospered, because the census that year listed a maid living at their residence. The railway station near the Nirenberg family home had opened earlier as a two-track surface station called South Midwood. The proximity of this station enabled Max to commute more easily to the shirt company's headquarters in Manhattan. Eventually Harry would join his father in the shirt business, but not before spending more than one and a half years in medical school.

In 1885, Marshall's great-grandmother on his mother's side, Fanny Landau, arrived in the United States at age 31. That same year the French ship *Isere* transported the Statue of Liberty's 300 copper pieces packed in 214 crates to America. The statue would welcome remnants of Marshall's ancestral family fleeing here for safety.

Fanny's husband, Wolf Rafelson, had immigrated to America from Russia a few years earlier. Although in the old country he may have been a rabbi or learned man, in his adopted country of America, he had to earn a living. He therefore had little time for prayer and contemplation and eventually owned a liquor store and a butcher shop. Together, Fanny and Wolf raised five children:—Lena, Mollie, Samuel, Jeanette, and Ralph. Lena would become Marshall's maternal grandmother.

Minerva Bykowsky, Marshall's mother-to be, was still in her teens when she met Harry Nirenberg. Her father, Samuel Bykowsky, came from Bialystock, Russia. He manufactured housedresses and aprons as the co-owner of the Empress Manufacturing Co. Minerva's sister, Sadie, recalled how her father loved opera and would take her as a child with him. When he first came to America, he would pay $2 for a ticket for standing room at the opera. Whereas Samuel displayed a very modern outlook (for example, supporting education for young women), his wife Lena seemed seemed less inclined to do so.

In July 1924, the *New York Times* announced the engagement of Harry Nirenberg and Minerva Bykowsky. The death of Minerva's father that same month cast a pall over the happy couple. The marriage took place at the Plaza Hotel, where the 28-year-old Harry took the 19-year-old Minerva as his bride. A year later, Harry's father, Max, also died. Harry and Minerva's first child, Joan, came in 1926, and Marshall followed a year later.

Marshall Meets the World

In 1927, indicators for the economic health of the nation seemed to be soaring. Writing about the preceding year, the *New York Times* intoned that the "outlook for money the present year continues promising. Despite the great expansion in credit for several years, economic conditions are so sound, accumulation of savings so great, reserve position so strong, that the business world has every reason to feel confident money rates will remain comfortable, on average hardly ruling higher than last year."[9]

By early 1929, people across the United States scrambled to get into the stock market. The profits seemed so assured that even many companies placed money in the stock market. And even more problematically, some banks placed customers' money in the stock market without their knowledge. With the stock market prices upward bound, everything seemed wonderful. When the great crash hit on October 24, 1929, these people were taken by surprise when stock prices plummeted. Vast numbers of people began selling their stocks. Margin calls for investors to repay their loans flooded the phone lines. People across the country watched as the numbers spit out spelled their economic demise. The ticker tape that displayed stock prices became so overwhelmed that it quickly fell behind. A crowd gathered outside of the New York Stock Exchange on Wall Street, stunned at the downturn. Rumors circulated of people committing suicide.[10]

The stock market downturn would continue for at least three years. By the time it ended, the average value of companies in the Dow Jones Industrials Average had dropped almost 90 percent. People found it increasingly difficult to get jobs. Farmers and rural residents felt the stock market crash as well—people and companies that used to buy food and other agricultural products no longer had the money to buy much of anything. The crash, along with other factors, produced an economic slowdown that lasted over 10 years and became known as "the Great Depression."[11]

Yet, Marshall later recalled:

In New York, we were upper middle-class people. I was not aware that there was a Depression when I was growing up. I think my father was very fortunate, so it didn't affect us. I had a happy life from the earliest time in Brooklyn. Later, we moved to Manhattan, overlooking the Hudson River, and then from there to Mount Vernon, New York. In Brooklyn and Mount Vernon we lived in houses. In Manhattan, we lived in an apartment. I went to public schools. There were books all over the house and my father subscribed to lots of magazines, so we came into contact with a lot of different things. I would read anything that was within reach.[12]

Marshall's sister Joan also remembered, "Marshall was my baby brother, but I was so young when he was born that I cannot ever remember a time without him. My baby brother—whom I have worried about, admired, cared for, looked up to, and always, always loved. He was, as a child, curious, gentle, and loving—and he stayed that way his entire life."[13]

Said Marshall:

I remember as a young child, sitting on the rug in the living room at my mother's feet. She was reading. I was putting together an erector set.

When I finished building I said with a great deal of excitement, "Mom, look what I've made!" She responded, "What is it Marshall?" At which point I said, "I don't know. What does it look like?" She looked at it and then at me and said, "Marshall, you have to begin with an idea of what you are going to create and then build it—not the other way around."[14]

However, she didn't realize that Marshall's mind worked differently from most. Sure, answers matter, but it's the process of discovery and the search for insight that thrilled him the most.[14]

In the summers, Marshall, his mother, and sister retreated from the heat of the city to a shaded cottage in the Catskill Mountains. Harry joined them on the weekends. Marshall vividly remembered the joy of collecting fossils and fishing with his father. Even the extreme nausea from seasickness and severe sunburn did not dim those memories. In the winter in New York, Marshall ice-skated; his parents took in an occasional play.[12]

Interspersed between visits to and from friends were trips abroad for Marshall's parents. When home, the family went to museums and to art galleries. Marshall roller-skated, played football and hockey on city streets, and took private piano lessons and violin lessons at the Juilliard School of Music. He soon dropped the violin lessons. "I considered the other Juilliard students so talented," said Marshall, "that I felt that I could not compare to them, so I just continued the piano lessons."[12]

That boyhood revelry would soon end in a crisis. In mid-winter in New York City on an outing with several other boys, Marshall became the target of a prank with life-threatening consequences. While watching some golden carp being taken out of a pool, one of the boys pushed him into the pool of ice-cold water. "I ran home as fast as I could," Marshall recalled. "By the time I got home, my pants were so frozen that even after I took them off, they stood up. I came down with rheumatic fever because of that."[12]

Marshall first developed a cold, with a seemingly minor sore throat. But in the 1930s, a bacterial infection that caused a sore throat could also damage the heart.[15–17] The occurrence of rheumatic fever made removal of tonsils, a potential source of sore throat, the most common operation in the United States after circumcision.[18] Although in the early 1930s, investigators knew that rheumatic fever occurred after a bacterial infection, it took decades for practicing doctors to accept their findings.[19] This confusion among medical experts and the absence of antibiotics for treatment did little for Marshall's parents, tormented by the thought that their son might become a lifelong invalid.

That Marshall now suffered from rheumatic fever proved an almost unbearable burden for Harry. Before Marshall was born, Harry had dropped out of medical school and had enlisted in the U.S. Army to fight in World War I. As a result, Harry knew well the dangers of rheumatic fever and feared the worst for his young son. Harry wanted to get away from the city, both to escape from the site of the trauma that had involved Marshall and possibly to arrive at a more rural, healthier environment. Therefore, Harry moved the family farther north to Mount Vernon. Harry might have felt that the "country air" of Mt. Vernon would be a welcome salve for Marshall's recovery. Whatever the reason, the family didn't stay long in Mount Vernon, for the phone books of that era make no listing of the Nirenbergs being there.

Throughout 1936, Marshall remained bedridden in Mount Vernon. Fear of the consequences from rheumatic fever rendered Marshall a semi-invalid.

During that interlude, he spent long hours alone, reading extensively. Marshall could not attend school, and so had to be tutored at home. Mel Shader, a younger boy, whose family had moved to Mount Vernon from Orlando, Florida, four years before, landed the tutoring assignment with the convalescing Marshall.[20]

Mel's tutoring paid an unexpected dividend. The Shaders introduced Marshall's family to two opportunities the Nirenbergs had previously never considered. First, the Shaders emphasized sunny Florida and the Orlando region, in particular, as a far better locale than Mount Vernon for the repair of Marshall's health. Second, the Shaders touted the money they made in dairy farming. In fact, said the Shaders, Mel's aunt and uncle owned the thriving College Park Dairy but just might be induced to sell it to the right buyer if a proper deal could be negotiated.[20]

The combined choice of Orlando and dairy farming greatly appealed to Harry, who must have feared for his son's life. A move to Florida seemed the best possible way to help Marshall recover. Harry's career in shirt manufacturing, while providing a solid living, might have grown unappealing to him. Perhaps he wanted to establish himself independent of his father, who had brought him into the shirt business and remained a somewhat dominant figure. Perhaps having lived his entire life in New York, Harry welcomed the change that a move to Florida would bring. Furthermore, he might have reasoned, he had partially completed medical school. If he already had the skills to handle human patients, how hard would it be to tend a herd of cows?

Accordingly, Harry set about to negotiate a deal to buy a dairy farm in Orlando. The deal would result in lifelong consequences for the entire family in ways that he could hardly imagine at the time. Perhaps he gave careful thought to the decision being made. Or possibly a sense of impulsiveness drove the changes being crafted. In the end, Harry cashed out his share of the shirt business to buy the farm. With this altruistic decision, Marshall's fortunes would ultimately rise while his father's fortune would fall.

2   A Land of Milk and Sunny

In 1937, Marshall and his family were about to find that New York City was as different from Orlando, Florida, as the moon is from the sun.

More than half a foot of snow fell in January as the Nirenberg family prepared to depart Mount Vernon for a whole new way of life in sunny Orlando, Florida. Bundled up in hats and long overcoats against the piercing, chilling wind, the family boarded The New York, Westchester and Boston Railway, an electric commuter railroad that ran from Mount Vernon to New York. The railroad was on its "last tracks," so-to-speak, having undergone bankruptcy proceedings in 1935.

Disembarking at the terminal station in the South Bronx, the family went underground to the New York subway system and rode down to the Pennsylvania Railroad Station at 31st Street and 8th Avenue. There, for perhaps one last time, 10-year-old Marshall would be overwhelmed, even in the grayness of the day, by the gargantuan structures that typified the most populous city in America. Unbelievable feats of engineering and mountains of steel, limestone, and brick throughout the city trumpeted each structure's contribution to the texture of the landscape.

By contrast, five- to seven-story structures called tenements dotted the city. The city's population of about seven million crammed into them.[1] Some 30 percent of the city's population at the time was, like Marshall's family, Jewish.

Small alleys in the back of the tenements held elevated line after line of fresh wash, flapping in the breeze while drying in the sun. Below the clothes lines, children played ball and whatever other games they could make up. On the streets, the city's mass of humanity flowed unceasingly over the crowded sidewalks like a river running over its bed. Store after store, sign over sign, greeted one as far as the eye could see along each busy thoroughfare.

At Pennsylvania Station, Marshall and his family boarded the *Orange Blossom Special* that would relieve them of this frenzy of humankind, the cacophony of city life, and the ubiquitous street odors one encountered in New York City. The *Orange Blossom Special* would be their one-way, magical carpet ride that would speed them instead to a bright, almost alien-type, Floridian world. The route was actually a combination of tracks borrowed from the Pennsylvania, Richmond, Fredericksburg & Potomac, and Seaboard Air Lines. "The *Orange Blossom Special* was a train with a mission: Ignore local traffic and intermediate stops; get those vacationing snowbirds [the Nirenberg family being one of the lone exceptions] from the frozen Northeast to sunny Florida as quickly as possible—in first class style."[2]

Operated only during the winter vacation season, this heavyweight train consisted of Pullman, dining, and baggage cars. On the train as it pulled out of Pennsylvania Station at 12:50 p.m., Marshall might have glimpsed scattered Hoovervilles. These migrant camps consisted of shanties and unemployed workers still in the throes of the Depression, which was slowly winding down.

It would take almost a full day of travel and about 900 miles of track to reach Wildwood, Florida. After stops in Newark and Trenton, New Jersey; Philadelphia, Pennsylvania; Wilmington, Delaware; Baltimore, Maryland; Washington, D.C.; and finally Richmond, Virginia, the train sped on through the South with no further stops until it reached Florida.

Arriving in Florida

When Marshall awoke the next morning, he found himself in an alien environment quite unlike New York. The life that lay in the future, here in Florida, would gradually awaken within Marshall largely dormant interests he had as he played in the gutters and streets of the city. Bright, warm sunlight streamed through the windows of the train. As Marshall stepped down onto the platform, the air was fragrant with the perfume of orange and grapefruit blossoms, gardenia flowers, and magnolia trees.

The family likely motored from Wildwood to nearby Orlando. There, they found a small city of some 35,000 people who made up the local populace. Each winter that number swelled by half again when northerners came down on the *Orange Blossom Special* to escape the harshness of winter and revel in the 31 lakes within Orlando's city limits and its 200 miles of brick-paved streets. The local economy depended heavily upon this flood of tourists and on local agriculture. Outside of the city, orange and grapefruit groves stretched for miles, alongside spreading fields of strawberries, celery, and other fresh vegetables.[3]

Unlike the tenements and skyscrapers of New York City, the architecture of Orlando varied from well-preserved two- to five-story brick business buildings and residences of the late nineteenth century. Many were resplendent with dormers, cupolas, stamped metal cornices or ornate structures of glazed tile embellished with chromium bands.[4] The Orlando Bank and Trust Company, dedicated in 1924, constituted one of the rare exceptions. The 10-story, 20th-century commercial style building, termed a skyscraper by the locals, stood at one of the most fashionable addresses in the city.[5]

Downtown Orlando at the time encompassed about eight blocks of buildings constructed from the 1880s. The medley of architectural styles ranged from Queen Anne and Twentieth Century Commercial to Beaux Arts, Manhattan Revival, Art Deco, and Art Moderne. Masonry composed nearly all of these buildings due to a series of fires in the late 1800s that destroyed many of the original wooden structures. The city, in response to the conflagration, had then enacted stringent building codes.[5]

The styles of homes reflected their owners' origins. Southerners preferred plantation houses with wide verandas and roof-high columns. English expatriates opted for brick English manor homes. Transplanted northerners chose the chaste New England cottage. Native Floridians preferred the flat-roof, tropical house. However, landscaping unified the diverse styles. Coral and golden flame vines and exotic flowering shrubs grew in nearly every yard.[4] In Orlando, social life centered on home invitations, clubs, musical and theater groups, and around the parks and recreational facilities. Nearby, Rollins College, Florida's oldest college, formed the center of Orlando's academic life; speakers of note, many leading artists of concert and stage, and nationally known educators smartly chose wintertime to come and exhibit their expertise.[4]

In January 1937, when the Nirenberg family arrived, social activity in the resort city of Orlando took a completely outdoor turn as central Florida experienced a midwinter heat wave. The unusually warm weather affected flowers and shrubs, causing them to burst into bloom a month ahead of schedule. Flame vine, named for an orange, mid-winter bloom that makes it look like a tongue of fire, bloomed profusely as did azaleas.[6]

The mild climate was just what the doctor ordered for Marshall. Free from frost for nearly nine months of the year, Orlando had neither snow nor extreme cold in the winter. Cool nights tempered the summer heat, rains made the grass grow, and dew appeared in the mornings to dampen it.[7]

The dairy Harry Nirenberg bought had its origins stretching back to the 1850s and 1860s. Drawn by opportunities to grow cotton and herd cattle, some Jewish families came with other pioneers to the "Old West" style town of Orlando. Records show that after the Civil War about 16 Jewish families lived in Orlando.[8] In the early part of the 20th century, one such family, the Wittensteins, bought land for a dairy farm in the northern part of today's College Park section of Orlando. The farm became bordered by Wittenstein Road.[9] The road, running east to west through Orlando, was bounded on the northwest, nearby Lake Daniel and Lake Sarah, and on the south central by Lake Silver.[10]

Harry Nirenberg perhaps never realized until he began operations just how difficult dairy farming would prove to be. Cows had to be milked twice daily, and the herd required constant attention day in and day out. Despite the hard physical labor that was also involved, Harry somehow found time to become active in one Jewish congregation and later help found another. Despite Harry's religious pursuits, friends of Marshall professed knowing nothing of his Jewish heritage, because Marshall never discussed it with them. Throughout the rest of his life, Marshall typically did not trumpet or press upon others his religious preferences and beliefs.[8,11]

Unlike many other residents of Orlando, the Nirenbergs found life far from idyllic. Over the years, Harry's business evolved through three phases. First came the dairy. Harry believed that Wittenstein had misled him about the ease and profitability of dairy ownership. Harry later diverted the milk into candy making about the time sugar rationing went into effect in World War II. Making candy with less sugar proved to be a serious handicap. Success finally came only in Harry's later years, when he converted the farm into commercial warehouses and rented the space to local companies. That final stage proved to be the most valuable of all. When Harry Nirenberg died, the insured value of his properties came to about $1.5 million in today's dollars.[12,13]

The dairy, however, formed the centerpiece of Marshall's life growing up in Orlando. He remembered:

We lived at the dairy: there was a house right on the grounds with orange trees and grapefruit trees. I picked pecans. It was right across the street from a 40-acre commercial orange grove, and there were lakes all around nearby. It was a very interesting place. One time a little plane landed in the pasture, and the pilot asked me, "Which way is Miami?" So I told him, and I also told him where he was, and he went off.[12]

Marshall worked at the dairy, shoveling fertilizer and clearing bitter-weed, which when eaten by the cows made their milk bitter. As Harry filled the silo with chopped up corn and stalks for the cows, Marshall worked inside, first watering the mixture and then walking around to tamp down and compress it. With time, the mixture fermented, becoming mildly alcoholic, and a favorite food of the cows.[12]

Orlando, the largest city in the interior of Florida, was a principality of vast contrasts and lakes. In the past millennia, the Florida peninsula lay beneath the sea, and marine deposits gave rise to a thick layer of limestone. When the limestone dissolved, giant sinkholes filled with water and formed the extensive lakes that Marshall eventually explored as a boy in Orlando. In 1937, Florida also contained 40 times more farm acreage alone—6 million acres—than the entire acreage of the city of New York. A small portion of that acreage was more than enough of a playground for young Marshall and his bike.[7,14]

Underground springs feeding many of the lakes helped moderate the climate throughout the year. Buildings often extended up to the edge of the lakes where water lapped the shore. Boulevards wound around the lakes, and the landscaped pathways offered shade with their live oaks, camphor trees, and a profusion of native and imported palms. Subtropical shrubs, citrus trees, and winter-blooming flowers filled many local gardens. The dull red brick-paved streets and the sparkling blue lakes contrasted against this background of evergreen foliage.[4] In addition to the lakes, Orlando housed swamps that would figure prominently in Marshall's interest in biology.

For fun, Marshall could enjoy the Orlando Drive-In Theater on South Orange Blossom Trail. Its sister theater, the Winter Park, touted the "first Florida showing" of Roy Rogers and Dale Evans in *My Pal Trigger* … "Filmed in Beautiful Trucolor." The Central Florida Exposition, Florida's oldest consecutive fair in Orlando, also provided some diversion. In 1937, the exposition grounds grew with the addition of a large new general exhibition building.

With its climate and location, Orlando soon became a mecca for the citrus industry. Initially, fruit from the first commercial citrus grove had to be hauled to the river and transported by boat to Charleston, South Carolina. As the citrus industry expanded, growers demanded an end to the long overland route. Consequently, the South Florida Railroad decided to extend its rail line to Orlando, which made Orlando more accessible and prominent. General Ulysses S. Grant turned the first spade of earth to start construction.[4]

In the 1920s, Orlando experienced the Florida Land Boom that consumed investors with dreams of big money and lured new citizens on each new train. The onset of the Great Depression turned those dreams into financial nightmares.[5]

Marshall did not seem particularly interested in the economic news of the day. Rather, Marshall much preferred the explorations of Orlando—a boyhood's dream—to the hard, smelly work on the dairy farm. In addition to the exotic flora and fauna to be discovered and observed, Orlando also had a fascinating history. Orlando, like that of other towns in central Florida, had become settled in the 1800s as an aftermath of the Seminole Wars, during which the native Seminoles were driven out of the Orlando area.[15,16] The initial site for Orlando came from its proximity to Fort Gatlin, established about 1837 because of the excellent water sources and the habitable highlands of the area.[4]

During the Civil War, when a Federal blockade stopped all shipments of cattle from Florida—part of the Southern rebellion—to Cuba, Orlando stockmen sold their beef to the Confederates, delivering it on the hoof to Charleston, South Carolina. When the Civil War ended, magazine articles described the fertile farming land and ideal climate of Orlando, and the city had another boom.[4] The widespread planting of citrus gave agriculture in central Florida an importance that drove the cattle to ranges farther south, and marked the passing of frontier life in the community.[4]

The rapid development of Orlando eventually stumbled badly shortly before Marshall arrived. In April, 1929, in an Orlando grove, a fruit fly infestation began that eventually extended north and northwest. State and local inspectors took to the field, quarantining large areas. Inspectors allowed no fruit to be shipped from the affected groves, and four companies of the National Guard had to be called out to enforce the ban. The fern and foliage industry also suffered because plants had to be washed clean of all dirt before they could be shipped—a condition that made survival unlikely. The government in October finally lifted the fruit fly ban, saving the industry from possible collapse. Neither the Florida citrus industry nor the rest of the nation's economy, however, would escape the onset of the Great Depression.[17]

But as a young boy blissfully unaware of many of these developments, Marshall's enthusiasm for his new life in Orlando could not be restrained. He remembered a totally wild area nearby of swamp and scrub pine. He could walk for about 20 miles without crossing a road or coming upon a house. After school, Marshall would hop on his bicycle and tramp around this newfound wonderland.[12]

For Marshall, Orlando was a natural paradise. The miles and miles of space gave Marshall an opportunity to wade and hunt, view a profusion of birds and plants and even catch an occasional cottonmouth moccasin, a poisonous water snake. Marshall would put the snake in a bag and bring it home. He recalled, "If my mother knew, she would have fainted. I remember one time she walked in the room and said, "What's that smell?" And I said, "What smell?" Then, I ... release[d] the snakes afterwards."[12]

Marshall had been interested in biology from the earliest he could remember. But from where did his passion spring? Marshall didn't know. But some of his earliest memories involved catching and pressing butterflies and winning nature awards at summer camp.[12]

Marshall's boyhood in Orlando coincided with the tapering off of consequences from the Great Depression. But echoes of the past economic downturn still reverberated in the community, as it did in the rest of the country. Orlando, like most other communities, had become depressed as tax delinquencies, business failures, and bank closings continued to pile up. Weeds had sprung up through the asphalt of streets of failed subdivisions. The inauguration of Franklin D. Roosevelt as president in 1933 led to the development of innovative, audacious, and controversial programs known collectively as the New Deal. The impact of these programs permanently altered the relationship between the national government and state and local communities. The federal government spent millions of dollars through grants-in-aid for hundreds of civic projects in Orlando and surrounding towns, to ease the suffering of people and the loss of jobs and property as a result of the Great Depression.[18]

About a year before Harry Nirenberg took over ownership of the College Park Dairy, signs of a recovery from the depression in Orlando became stronger. In December 1935, an automobile show was held for the first time in several years. Deposits at the city's three banks showed more than a 50 percent increase. Bell Telephone had a 15 percent increase in patrons, and other utilities reported similar gains. A Festival of Progress featuring a huge parade in 1936 celebrated these signs of improvement. Statewide, Orlando ranked second only to Miami in per capita retail sales. Building permits exceeded a million dollars for the first time since 1928. At least one new housing subdivision and several new businesses opened.[19]

As the Nirenberg family settled into their new life at the dairy, utility services and school registrations began setting new records. Construction of hundreds of new residential homes moved to completion, some costing more than $70,000. The Chamber of Commerce estimated the city's permanent population had that year increased by 10,000; the influx of visitors totaled 29,000. The Southern Bell Telephone Co. installed hundreds more telephones, Eastern Air Lines began offering direct express service to New York and Chicago, and railroads expanded their services to and from Orlando.[20]

Up to this point, Marshall's interest in biology had been largely self-taught. That would greatly change with the expansion of the local airport and the entry of the United States into World War II. Municipal Airport, proudly completed in 1928, had fallen into such disrepair that the government threatened to discontinue the mail flights that landed there. To prevent that from happening, the city agreed to expand and improve the airport.[21] The changes brought an almost immediate response from commercial airlines and regular flights ensued. With the start of World War II, the Army Air Corps chose the airport as its headquarters.

These developments profoundly affected Marshall. During World War II, the Army brought in professional biologists to teach a jungle survival course for pilots going to the South Pacific. As part of local outreach efforts, the biologists took Marshall and his friends, Jim Pittman and Jim Boyles, on field trips and overnight camping trips around the region. Marshall also met other biologists who passed through Orlando, including Roger Tory Peterson, a noted naturalist and ornithologist.[12] Jim Pittman, who became a physician, later said, "I think that encounter with those *real biologists* was a critical point in making us what we became and are today."[22]

Letting his enthusiasm get away, Marshall once needed the help of one of the biologists, George Sutton. A game warden had caught Marshall shooting birds without a license and took him to a judge. Somehow Sutton, back in Ohio, heard about the incident. Sutton sent the judge a telegram telling him that Marshall was collecting specimen birds for the jungle survival course. So Marshall was let off with just a warning.[12]

Pittman, who had a car, also drove with Marshall around Central Florida. Despite the war and the rationing of gasoline, Pittman's father got an extra ration of gasoline because of his essential business. Jim and Marshall shared a mutual love of natural history and used the car for field trips. Once in a cave near Tampa, the two boys found the floor littered with large fossils, and fossil bones sticking out from the walls. One turned out to be the skull of a long-extinct saber-tooth tiger. In the summer, Marshall would also join the Pittman family at their lake cottage, where the two friends would swim and canoe together. Marshall greatly admired Jim Pittman. "[He] was a terrific boy," said Marshall, "... the kind of boy that every other boy wished he could be like. He was sort of a natural leader and had a wonderful ability to talk to people. ... He made friends wherever he went."[12]

These boyish adventures drove Marshall's interest in biology during a key formative phase of his life. The contact with professional biologists and the exposure to wildlife gave Marshall invaluable hands-on experience. The year of relative solitude in Mount Vernon when he recuperated from rheumatic fever had also made Marshall an avid reader. Other boys like him back in New York might fantasize about adventures in the wild and read about life in books. But Marshall didn't have to imagine the sights, sounds,

and odors of life outdoors. He now lived the dream, and it made a deep and lasting impression.

While Marshall reveled in the vast playground that Orlando offered him, his father labored under the heavy yoke of running the dairy. He might well have expected a grateful Marshall to help lift the burden from his aching shoulders. Yet, at the same time, he likely felt constrained from imposing too much hard labor on a boy still recovering from the effects of rheumatic fever. The net result may have been Harry's resentment toward Marshall. As Marshall's health improved, he became increasingly disinterested in following in his father's steps in the dairy.

Jim Boyles, Marshall's boyhood friend, recalled the first time he met Marshall's father, "[Marshall's] father was not friendly. ... I couldn't tell whether he disliked me, or whether he was angry at Marshall. ... At that time, my impression was he was angry at Marshall for not working, but dilly-dallying around—playing around collecting spiders and snakes."[11]

Marshall's mother seemed similarly disenchanted with her removal from New York where she had lived all of her young life. Minerva was very sociable and had friends and family in the New York area, so adjusting to life on a dairy farm was a major change for her. She had never worked for money until Harry moved into the candy business. To help out, Minerva made fudge that stores in Orlando sold—a confection that earned kudos from the local populace. During World War II, Minerva studied structural drawing, learning how to draw machine parts in three dimensions for plans for assembly of machines. But Minerva never used whatever she had learned in the course.[12] Perhaps Harry felt that if Minerva had to have a paying job doing mechanical drawings, it would highlight to the community his struggles to support a family. He could, however, rationalize her making and selling fudge as a homemaker's "hobby."

Life for the Nirenberg family included other challenges that may have led to Marshall becoming the somewhat withdrawn and very private person he remained for the rest of his life. The Nirenberg family encountered problems endemic to southern culture, problems faced less frequently in the North. The presence of the Ku Klux Klan was one. The segregation of blacks was another. In the North, whether in Brooklyn or Mount Vernon, the family had been part of large and vibrant Jewish communities. In Orlando, to a large extent, they existed in isolation with few friends and no family in the immediate area.

Marshall's ancestors had come to America to escape the hatred and bigotry encountered in Eastern Europe. Now their descendants in Orlando faced a similar situation. The Ku Klux Klan, whose members hated Jews as well as Catholics and blacks, found its most powerful klaverns (local branches) in Orlando and a few other cities in Florida.[23] *The Birth of a Nation*, a catalyst for the reappearance of the Ku Klux Klan, caused racial trouble everywhere the movie played. In Orlando, the film broke all attendance records at the Grand Theater.[24]

Racism in Florida persisted throughout Marshall's teenage years and beyond. Orlando remained the last city in Florida to retain an all-white voting primary, despite a ruling by the Supreme Court banning the practice.[25] During the years Marshall lived in Orlando, the area continued to be wracked with racially motivated violence. Shootings and lynchings of blacks occurred. The owner of an apartment complex, for example, applied for rezoning for black occupancy. The complex received a dynamite blast in response. The stillness of another night was shattered by the explosion of a small Creamette Frozen Custard Stand that refused to separately serve whites and blacks.[26]

Segregated newspapers printed segregated news. The nearby city of Sanford refused to allow Jackie Robinson, then active on a Brooklyn Dodgers farm team, to take the field with white players. White and black criminals could not be hung on the same gallows or even at the same time of the day. Buses and other forms of mass transportation as well as their stations segregated passengers by race. Some places denied blacks the right to drive on main streets or to park along any streets. Swimming pools, even beaches, opened for whites only. Signs on restrooms and drinking fountains kept the races separated. The facilities for blacks were often in inferior condition.[24]

No evidence exists that the Klan directly intimidated or attacked the Nirenberg family, who were ensconced in their little farmhouse at the College Park Dairy. But surely the existence of the Klan and news of its frequent activities likely hung over the family like a dark cloud. This may account, at least in part, for the strong sense of conscience and social responsibility Marshall exhibited throughout his life. Similarly, Marshall's sister Joan, despite the personal danger, became active in the civil rights movement when she lived in Alabama.

The family experienced other difficulties as well. In addition to the often back-breaking work of the dairy, Harry Nirenberg also faced unexpectedly the myriad complications of the milk industry. Dairy farmers often found themselves at the mercy of the larger milk processors. Processors set prices for the milk they purchased. If the farmers didn't like it, they could try to sell their milk elsewhere. Often farmers could not and ended up in frustration, dumping the milk from the cans onto the dirt of their dairies.

When the Great Depression hit, demand for milk dropped sharply. The programs set up to regulate milk prices broke down. The government eventually stepped in to stabilize the market and help equalize the market power of dairy farmers with milk processors. Ensuring that consumers had adequate and dependable supplies of milk at reasonable prices also drove government action. Eventually, during World War II, demand increased for farm commodities including milk. Shifts in agreements made between farmers and processors and continued readjustment of milk prices complicated the business of dairy farming.[27]

Marshall avoided these milk matters and focused on academics. He found school in Florida to be about a year behind the New York curriculum. In Orlando High School, he took college preparatory courses in chemistry, physics, mathematics, algebra, geometry, English, literature, German, and Spanish. Marshall remembered that even before news of the atom bomb leaked out, his chemistry teacher had discussed the immense potential of atomic energy. He said, Marshall recalled, "that nobody thus far had succeeded in making it. Then he looked at the class—I thought he looked at me—and said, 'Maybe one of you will find the answer to that.' That kind of raised goose pimples on me!"[12]

In the 1940s, students could accelerate through high school and start college early. Close to graduating, Marshall feared being drafted when he celebrated his 17th birthday. He got his father's consent to join the Merchant Marine. He thought life would be much more exciting in that service. Later, he realized the loss of ships of the Merchant Marine from enemy torpedoes could have cost him his life. The issue became moot when the Merchant Marine rejected Marshall on account of his rheumatic fever.

So rather than going off to war, Marshall decided to go off to college.[12]

3   Drifting Away

Unlike the experiences of other Nobel Laureates when they were younger, Marshall failed to impress his boyhood teachers or college professors. In contrast, James Watson, who shared the Nobel Prize for the discovery of the structure of DNA, received a tuition scholarship to the University of Chicago at the age of 15. He earned his PhD in zoology when he had just turned 22.

Richard Feynman, the Nobel-winning physicist, won the New York University Math Championship in his last year of high school. His high score both shocked the judges and clearly separated him from the other competitors. Feynman went on to graduate from the Massachusetts Institute of Technology. He then achieved perfect math and physics scores on the entrance exams for graduate school at Princeton University—an unprecedented feat.

Both Feynman and Watson would later become members of the RNA Tie Club and would compete against Marshall for discovery of the genetic code.

Marshall garnered no such early academic achievements. At Orlando High School, he reinforced his budding interest in science with chemistry, physics, algebra, and calculus. He graduated high school in 1945, however, with America still in the throes of World War II. Marshall certainly had reason to pause at one of the several crossroads of life he would encounter over the next seven decades.

Of course, he could contemplate going to college. But how would Marshall decide which college to attend? As one study of college choice noted: "In the 1930s, students appeared to make choices determined by vague notions of college reputation, facilities and personal values. .... In general, students had little interest in doing extensive research on the colleges and universities they were considering. ... In addition, the societal norms and values of the times further constrained the college-choice process for many students." [1] The behavior of these students could be explained by the lack of resources that they otherwise needed to make more informed decisions. In 1940, the country lacked a clearinghouse or central educational bureau to inform students about the numerous colleges and universities. This left students and parents with little to rely on except institutionally produced promotional brochures, pictures and catalogs of varying quality. This material offered little in the way of substance or a basis for comparing one institution with another.[1]

But Marshall's choice of college proved more problematic than just the lack of a suitable college guide. Education held an exalted place in the lives of his family. Marshall's father had made it through almost two years of medical school at Cornell.

Marshall's older sister, Joan, had opted to attend college out of state at the University of Alabama. Her decision arose from the refusal of the University of Florida at the time to admit women. As a male, Marshall faced no such obstacle. He made a pragmatic decision to attend the University of Florida. His family had little money, but as an in-state student at the University of Florida he would not have to pay tuition. He would, however, have to pay a "registration fee" of $50 each semester to cover contingencies, construction and rehabilitation of buildings, infirmary care, student activities, and use of the swimming pool.[2]

Marshall might have been further deterred in his college choices by the possible quotas that many schools had at the time for admittance of Jewish students. Alvin and Rodney Blocker, two brothers who grew up with Marshall in Orlando, both eventually made their way through medical school. Yet, they both recalled, "There were lots of qualified people who never seemed to get into a school, or who had great difficulty getting into a school. Now the whole business of quota is … shrouded in all sorts of mystery. … But we certainly all felt that there was a quota, so far as Jewish students were concerned."[3]

During World War II, for young men fortunate enough to remain at home, college remained the most likely prospect at that time. One of Marshall's schoolmates in high school noted, "If you scored in the upper five percentile of everybody that took the entrance exam … they let you become a freshman at the University of Florida, and when you finished your freshmen year, they gave you your high school diploma."[4] And so Marshall started college at the University of Florida in Gainesville in the second semester of his senior year in high school. The war made it possible for him to accelerate his education.

The University of Florida became part of the land-grant college system set up during Abraham Lincoln's tenure as president. As one writer has noted:

The goal of land-grant colleges was, among other things, to democratize this [American] system of [higher] education: early supporters of such schools, writes historian Allan Nevins, believed that "no restrictions of class, or fortune, or sex, or geographical position—no restrictions whatsoever— should operate." The same went for race. [Justin Smith] Morrill [who introduced the act] emphasized that African-Americans and Native Americans deserved schooling too.[5]

The irony, of course, lay in the fact that when Marshall entered college, the University of Florida admitted neither women nor blacks. The university first admitted women in 1947; equal higher education for blacks had to wait 11 years more, well after Marshall had left.[6]

During the 1940s, the University of Florida did not rank as one of the outstanding universities in the United States. Certainly, the school did not merit the same attention and prestige that MIT or the University of Chicago received. In 1940, Charles Lovejoy did a school ranking based on the publication, *Who's Who*, using the entries for 1937–1940. This publication touted contemporary prominent people of the time. In doing so, it reverted back to the earlier emphasis on wealth and prestige that presaged college attendance. Lovejoy determined from the *Who's Who* the "absolute number of entries" of individuals that graduated from each institution of higher education. He used the entries as an indirect means of ranking the relative worth of those institutions. Not surprisingly, several private Ivy-League institutions, such as Harvard, Yale, Columbia, and Princeton, topped the list. Several state universities did as well: Cornell, the University of Michigan, University of Wisconsin, and the University of California, Berkeley. The University of Florida failed to make the cut.[7]

Marshall began college when unemployment in America rested at 1.9 percent, and he could write home for the cost of a 3-cent first-class stamp. The Atomic Age had begun a few months earlier when the first atomic bomb had been tested at Alamogordo, New Mexico; the Cold War loomed ahead in the future.

The University of Florida in Gainesville welcomed in-state students like Marshall, and he probably did not apply elsewhere. His decision to attend the university in Gainesville also centered on remaining in a warm environment for his health and staying close to home. Gainesville resided only a little over 100 miles from Orlando. Situated within an hour's drive from both the Atlantic and Gulf coasts, the university's setting provided Marshall with abundant opportunities for recreation. The climate was perfect for his health as well. It featured a mild winter, a pleasant spring and fall, along with a hot, humid summer for four months.

Off to College

Marshall began his studies in the winter of 1945. In addition to Biological World and General Chemistry, his courses included Reading/Speaking/Writing, First Year Infantry, and Man's Social World. The following semesters saw a mix of some biology and chemistry and further humanities courses. Marshall generally earned A's and B's except for three courses: Analytical Chemistry taken in the summer of 1946, Organic Chemistry, and First Year Infantry, each of which generated a grade of C. At the end of the fall 1946 semester, Marshall received an associate of arts degree.

He returned for the winter semester of 1947 and embarked on earning a bachelor of science degree. In these higher level courses, Marshall did not fare quite as well as before. Lecturers droned on in large lecture halls filled not just with 20-year olds like Marshall but with men recently returned from fighting in World War II. These veterans savored the rewards of victories and freedom by completing their educations under the G.I. Bill of Rights.

In the next four semesters, Marshall earned 10 C's and 3 D's, although the latter grades revolved around his study of German. Marshall's graduation on July 24, 1948, came with a lackluster grade point average of just 2.32 for his final two years.

Significantly, Marshall tasted freedom at college. He remained far removed from the hard, sweaty labor of the dairy and the muck that stuck to his shoes as he walked through the fields. Somewhat reserved but likable, Marshall joined Pi Lambda Phi, a social fraternity on campus that had its own fraternity house. Marshall first lived on the university campus in a dormitory and later in the fraternity house. Recalls Stanley Becker, "When I went to school there, it cost 75 dollars a semester [probably for various fees] plus thirty dollars a semester for used books, and a dollar a day for three meals, a dollar a day to live in the fraternity house."[4]

At one point, Marshall stated that his fellow fraternity brothers elected him to be the social chairman of the group. This meant time away from his studies to organize parties. Perhaps some of the distractions of fraternity life adversely affected Marshall's ability to concentrate on his studies. A schoolmate from Orlando at the time remembers, "I liked Marshall; he was a very likeable guy. Anybody that would meet him would certainly like him and immediately realize that he was a little more intelligent than your average guy."[4] Jim Boyles, a childhood friend, described the Marshall he knew: "He was a nice, sweet, boy. Very kind hearted, likeable, quiet. He was just a—you know, he was one of those people that you're glad you knew."[8]

These memories of Marshall contrast with those of others who also knew him. One of his fraternity brothers at the University of Florida recalled, "He was a very laid-back guy. He, of course, was into his entomology and, as I remember Marshall, he always had a jar of lizards or bugs or something that he was watching or dissecting. ... I don't recall that he was particularly socially oriented. ... He would stay to himself more. ... Probably a little below the average guy his age as far as social activity goes."[9] These comments from a fraternity brother make Marshall's election as social chairman somewhat surprising.

Although Marshall entered the university in 1945, it took him only three years to graduate since he had been able to take college level courses while still in high school. During his college years, Marshall worked as a teaching assistant, which earned him some additional spending money. An undergraduate teaching assistantship was uncommon. Marshall recalled, "There weren't that many people attending the University of Florida then. Because of the war very few people were there, only 500 or 600. ... I think the courses I took in the biology department had an influence, and I taught comparative anatomy and some other courses that had an influence. I made friends with the faculty. I was working in the biology department; so I knew the professors who worked there."[10]

Marshall's remembered his college days fondly: "It was a marvelous experience. It was all boys. It was a monastic school at that time; now it's coeducational. There was a great sense of freedom. Working and teaching there made life just wonderful because I could keep my own hours."[10]

"My hours, though, were always terrible. I always worked at night. I liked to work at night, and I hated to get up in the morning. So there was nobody to tell me to get up and nobody telling me to go to sleep—which I really liked. I liked learning, and so I really enjoyed college very, very much."[10]

Marshall returned to the dairy farm and, in between mucking in the fields and milking in the barn, spent two more years contemplating his life and future. Deciding that becoming a dairy farmer suited him no better than it had his father, Marshall returned to the University of Florida to pursue the love of biology that living in Orlando had ignited within him. "During that period," Marshall explained," my father had this candy factory, and I wasn't sure what I was going to do with my life. So I became a salesman for the candy factory products. I traveled all around the state selling candy during that time. I didn't like it; so I went back to graduate school."[10]

Despite his low grade point average as an undergraduate, the University of Florida welcomed Marshall back and admitted him into the master's program in zoology. Here, Marshall got his first taste of biochemistry and, perhaps relishing the challenge of a graduate program, excelled. Admitted in the winter of 1950, Marshall graduated on February 2, 1952, with an election to Phi Beta Kappa and an almost perfect scholastic record. While Marshall appeared to have turned a corner insofar as grade attainment, his record as a PhD student later would suggest otherwise.

Later in life, Marshall said he relished the challenge of working on "cutting-edge" science. Yet, the choices he made while at the University of Florida, and later as a graduate student at the University of Michigan, suggest he did not do that while still a student. From 1950 to 1952, Marshall helped pay his way through the zoology graduate program by working with radioactive materials as a research associate in the Nutrition Laboratory at the University of Florida. This became Marshall's first exposure to biochemistry, the field that would prove to be the epitome of his scientific career.

The primitive counter then in use for measuring radioactivity had a probe that went into the liquid sample to be counted. After measuring the radioactivity for a set amount of time, Marshall had to move the probe to the next vial with a sample. By working with two different counters, Marshall managed to double the output of data each session. Then he did all of the calculations for each radioactive sample to quantify the results. Marshall liked doing the experiments and enjoyed the people with whom he worked. As an introduction to biochemistry, the experience in the Nutrition Laboratory could not have been better. Marshall's name appeared for the first time in a published scientific paper that used radioactivity to trace biological changes in the tissues of hens laying eggs.

The use of radioactive isotopes for scientific studies in biochemistry had exploded after the end of World II in 1945. The Nutrition Laboratory became one of the first to use radioactively labeled compounds to trace what happened to them in the bodies of animals. Marshall's work there ended in 1952. The next year, President Dwight D. Eisenhower appeared before the United Nations. In his Atoms for Peace speech, he proposed the expanded use of radioactivity for peaceful purposes. While scientifically valuable, Eisenhower hoped this strategy would also help offset the destructive use of radioactivity caused by the atom bomb during the war on Japan.

Using radioactivity in biological studies defined a new frontier of biochemistry. Marshall seemed well positioned to take advantage of this new advance through his work in the Nutrition Laboratory. But Marshall may not have fully appreciated the new opportunity radioactivity presented. From the winter semester of 1950 through the fall of 1951, Marshall did coursework for his master's degree in zoology. His early work with radioactivity whetted his appetite for biochemistry, a field in which he would later cement his reputation with the genetic code. But those events lay in the distant future.

Instead, Marshall now opted to catalog flies. In selecting a research topic for his thesis, Marshall made a curious choice. Research on biological subjects can be divided into two broad classes: research that is based simply on observation versus research that is driven by the making and testing of a hypothesis. Observation means just that: the investigator observes and reports on a phenomenon. The success of the project entails minimal risk. In hypothesis-driven research, the researcher first devises an idea that predicts some new phenomenon from the known facts. Then the researcher tests that idea experimentally and gathers hard data to confirm or deny the hypothesis. The idea may or may not work out.

So devising a hypothesis is akin to playing Russian roulette with one's professional career. Hypothesis-driven research involves greater risk because one cannot be certain the idea is correct. Of course, one may gather greater professional reward if the hypothesis is correct, so the stakes surrounding hypothesis-driven research are much higher. Consequently, observational science is not as highly regarded as hypothesis-driven studies.

Marshall might have chosen a problem in which radioisotopes could have been used to test a hypothesis. For example, he might have wondered how chickens make hemoglobin, which is responsible for the red color of blood. Marshall might then have used a radioactive agent to confirm or deny his idea. Instead he opted for an observational thesis project. Marshall recalled:

Lewis Berner was my mentor for my master's thesis in the biology department. He … [was] … a systematic entomologist, a very nice person. George Davis was head of the Nutrition Lab, and Ray Shirley was a biochemist working in the Nutrition Lab, and the person with whom I worked the most and who directed my work in the Nutrition Lab. That was my first exposure to biochemistry. There were no courses in biochemistry offered at that time; so it opened up a new field which I thought I would really enjoy doing.[10]

Marshall chose to work with Berner on the caddis flies of Alachua County. At the time, of 63 species of caddis flies previously found in Florida, 38 species came from Alachua County. Caddis flies are a group of generally overlooked, mostly dull brownish, moth-like insects found mainly near fresh water. They are medium-sized insects with bristle-like and often long antennae. Their generally hairy wings are held tent like over their bodies when at rest. Most caddis organisms rest a lot because they are weak fliers.

Marshall collected caddis flies as the basis for his master's thesis. He watched them build complicated houses from pieces of vegetation and saw them cement grains of sand as if to decorate the outside of the houses. He found he could collect the caddis flies by hanging a rope between two trees, with a white sheet slung over it, and a gasoline lantern in front. The flies would land on the sheet, where Marshall then collected them.[10]

Marshall believed that unlike northern regions, caddis flies in Florida were, for the most part, *not* a major food source for fish or other aquatic creatures. Caddis flies were, however, an important indicator of water quality. Many forms of caddis flies found in Floridian streams had an extremely low tolerance for polluted water. Just one particular species of caddis fly could tolerate it. Comparing the number of pollution-tolerant to pollution-intolerant flies gave an indication of how badly damaged a particular stream might be.

Marshall even managed to inject some excitement into his research on the flies. He brought dates along with him when he went out to collect caddis flies. The girls seemed to put up with his activities, although they did not say how much they enjoyed it.[10]

Marshall's study of caddis flies resembled his youthful study and collection of spiders for the American Museum of Natural History in New York City. On a family visit to New York, as a teenager, Marshall managed to establish a relationship with the museum's curator when he shared some specimens he'd brought with him. The museum provided Marshall with materials for collecting more specimens. Thus began an arrangement by which Marshall periodically sent specimens to the museum. (Marshall believed that the museum had actually named a rare spider after him. They called it the "Marshall spider." However, the museum today has no record of any such specimen.[11])

Marshall's selection of caddis flies incurred little risk. Caddis flies were already well-known in Alachua County. Marshall simply focused on describing the different species. Granted, Marshall himself collected 10,000 specimens and examined 800 others collected by collaborators. But had he only collected half or less of that number, it would not have mattered. With the completion and acceptance by his committee of his research, Marshall left the university once more. He would not return for another 20 years.

Marshall now had to decide on what to do next. He considered going into medicine. His close friend, Jim Pittman, had already done so. Pittman would later become an academic at the University of Alabama, where he sought to get Marshall a faculty position. But the chairman of the biochemistry department at that time would not consider appointing a Jew.[10]

The Higher Education of Another Nirenberg

In entering medicine, Marshall would have followed a choice his father made earlier. Marshall's father, Harry Edward Nirenberg, had planned to become a doctor after entering Cornell University in the fall of 1916.

Harry proved to be a student of exceptional ability who quickly grasped the opportunities offered. Although he entered a four-year program in 1916, he must have received considerable advanced standing. After only two years, Harry graduated from Cornell College in 1918 with a bachelor of arts degree. Harry had already been admitted to Cornell University Medical College in September 1917. Taking advantage of a special provision at Cornell, in the fall of 1917, Harry substituted a first year in medical school for his senior year in college.

In March 1918, Harry left Cornell and instead enlisted in the Reserve Corps of the U.S. Army. World War I was raging, and Harry wanted to volunteer. His enlistment papers described him as 5 feet 8½ inches tall, with a medium build, brown hair, and blue eyes. He began as a private in the medical section of the Army and was required to remain for four years. However, the war's end on November 11, 1918, shortened his Army service to less than a year, and he was released from the Army with the rank of captain. He never returned to Cornell to finish medical school.

There could have been several reasons why Harry left medical school for good. He may have found the program in New York less to his liking. Coursework no longer focused on the basic sciences as it had at Ithaca but now involved clinical work and patients.

Harry may have also recognized the limits of medicine in the early part of the 20th century. Immigrants, in particular, filled the streets of New York. Many arrived almost penniless to the land of opportunity and ended up living in filth and squalor. How could a doctor alleviate disease under such conditions? And even if a doctor wanted to help, what could he or she do? No antibiotics, for example, existed at the time for treating infectious diseases.

Whatever the reason for his seemingly impulsive decision to drop out of medical school, Harry wanted something completely different. Joan, Marshall's older sister, remembered, "My aunt Sadie, my mother's sister, stated that when my father got out of the service, he didn't want to go back to school. He wanted to join the shirt business with his father, Max. But his father told him first to get a job, be successful, and then he would take him into the business.[12]

Some family members think that Harry left medical school as the result of meeting Minerva Bykowsky, who would become his wife. Perhaps Harry did not want to delay raising a family though it certainly seemed that the affluence of Harry and Minerva's families would have kept the young couple financially secure. As evidence of this, their nuptials took place at the Plaza Hotel, one of the fanciest hotels in New York City. Harry had enough money to go to Cornell and then on to medical school, and Marshall and his sister, Joan, had been repeatedly told, Minerva had graduated from Barnard College. However, there is no record of Minerva actually going to Barnard or other colleges in New York City.[13–15]

Marshall Moves On

Although believing his father later regretted dropping out of medical school, Marshall faced different circumstances when he contemplated his future. His parents struggled to make a decent living on the dairy farm, and they had no spare funds to support further education for Marshall. Harry seemingly squelched any plans Marshall had entertained to become a doctor. Harry's partial medical training gave him good reason to worry almost obsessively over his son's health. Harry knew from first-hand experience that medicine was a hard and stressful profession—especially in the first half of the 20th century. Doctors made house calls at all hours of the day and night. Doctors found few if any "normal" days that other professionals enjoyed. Infectious diseases like tuberculosis, rheumatic fever, and pneumonia threatened the lives not only of patients but the doctors who treated them. Doctors carried little black bags that held their stethoscopes, blood pressure cuffs, and thermometers, but little else to fight disease.

Had the move to Orlando "cured" Marshall of his rheumatic fever? Or had Marshall's heart been somehow affected by the infection? One could never be certain. Remnants of the disease could still persist. So the field of medicine for Marshall, his father believed, might be dangerous to his health.

Marshall might have worked at the dairy. But he knew all too well what life and work on the dairy farm entailed. Even in high school, he had arisen at 5:00 a.m. in the morning to muck the stalls of the family farm. It was not the hard work that made Marshall averse to making milk his life's pursuit. It was the routine of farm life—predictable, unexciting, and not very stimulating.

So that left science. Marshall had an early and avid interest in biology. That innate interest in science had been fully awakened by the move to Orlando.

Yet even as a teenager, Marshall's actions were unique. After all, how many teens are asked to contribute insect specimens to a world-famous natural history museum? If Marshall wanted to make a living as a scientist, he had two choices. One involved getting a job in a laboratory working for someone else. But Marshall, like his father before him, showed a strong sense of independence. Working for someone else was not a trait exhibited by men in his family, many of whom had independently carved out successful niches in businesses. Besides, Marshall enjoyed school, so why not continue on to another graduate degree in the sciences? As a 25-year-old man, Marshall had outgrown tramping the swamps of Orlando for flies, snakes, and spiders. Now Marshall prepared to embark on the trip of a lifetime.

Marshall, at 25 years of age, awoke one morning to a long-delayed decision that would carry him light years away from Orlando, Florida. Always the dutiful son, he had had stayed close to home, graduating from the University of Florida in Gainesville with multiple degrees. Perhaps it was time to move on. He had been willing to undertake his college education in the South, but his future seemed positioned well north of Florida's borders.

Perhaps, Marshall thought, schools up north might be more challenging and jobs more plentiful. The difficulties his father continually faced become an object lesson Marshall wished to avoid. Securing a job, lifelong if possible, would become one of his highest priorities. His family's roots still remained deep in New York. Marshall turned his back on sunny Orlando and headed up north.

Marshall may have decided that his master of science degree failed to put sufficient distance between himself and life on the farm. Besides, Marshall loved science, reveled in science, thought of little else but science, and perhaps dreamed of becoming a scientist. Maybe a PhD program far from the environs of Florida would be most beneficial. But where to go? Details of how Marshall chose graduate programs are lost in the shifting strands of memory. Likely, Marshall turned for advice to several scientists whom he knew and admired.

Marshall's graduate work credits several individuals for help with his caddis flies research. He mentions Donald Gordon Denning of the University of Wisconsin as one. Perhaps coincidence, perhaps not, Marshall applied to the University of Wisconsin. James Speed Rogers's name also appears, who at the time worked at the University of Michigan. Not surprisingly, Marshall also applied to the University of Michigan. As both men were role models for the young zoologist, Marshall held them in high regard, and likely queried them about departments at their respective institutions.

Yet, Denning and Rogers's role in his decision making also had limitations. Based on his experience with biochemistry in the Nutrition Laboratory in Florida, Marshall opted not for zoology but instead for biochemistry departments. Marshall also applied to Duke University's department of biochemistry, then headed by Philip Handler, who would become the president of the prestigious National Academy of Sciences in Washington, D.C., 17 years later. Handler had made his reputation in the biochemistry of nutrition, and George K. Davis and Ray Shirley were the two biochemical nutritionists under whom Marshall worked in the Nutrition Laboratory. Davis and Shirley had set out to be the first to use radioactivity to trace how large domestic animals use nutrients.

In deciding where to go next, Marshall possibly heard Handler's name prominently mentioned in conversations in the Nutrition Laboratory. Nevertheless, the biochemistry department at Duke, with only five professors, was relatively small. Although Duke accepted Marshall, it did not offer him financial aid. Marshall, with little, if any, money available from his family, scratched Duke University off his list.

It seems ironic that Marshall considered going to either Michigan or Wisconsin, given that 15 years earlier his family had fled to the warmth of Orlando's balmy 72° average temperatures just to safeguard his health. The average year-round temperature for Madison, Wisconsin, is just 45°F, whereas that for Ann Arbor, Michigan is slightly higher at 50°F. Marshall claimed that he chose the University of Michigan because he mistakenly thought Michigan enjoyed warmer weather than Wisconsin. The difference was miniscule.

In retrospect, Marshall's consideration of distant, cold locales may have been his reaction to being treated like an invalid, for Marshall still had remnants of rheumatic fever. Alternatively, Marshall may have been engaging in a subtle but youthful rebellion against what he might have perceived to be an overly protective family.

When Marshall was applying to schools, the department of biochemistry at Wisconsin was older and more accomplished than the one at Michigan. The Wisconsin department traced its roots back to 1883. Research by the department faculty had already helped a host of public health advances, ranging from enhancing milk quality and producing penicillin on a large scale to discovering the vitamin A and the vitamin B complexes; isolating vitamin B6 derivatives; eradicating rickets with vitamin D; making essential niacin (vitamin B3) available to treat deficiencies; treating nutritional anemia; discovering dicumarol, one of the most clinically important "blood thinners"; and helping conceive the artificial insemination industry.

The Michigan biochemistry department had begun almost 40 years later in the 1920s. The department resided in the medical school and traced its roots back to a course in urine analysis that began in the 1860s. When Marshall arrived in 1952, Howard Bishop Lewis had begun celebrating 30 years as chairman. But during Lewis's long tenure, the department had made few strides in moving from physiological chemistry to the more modern outlook of biochemistry. Despite its much later start, the department already found itself outdated.

Marshall entered on less than stellar terms. The university admitted him with some misgivings, and the department of biochemistry promptly placed him on probation. The department's action may have reflected concern whether his graduation from a southern school, his undistinguished grade point average, and his degrees in zoology would hinder successful completion of the PhD biochemistry program. Why did the university then accept him at all? The reason may be that the weak biochemistry department at the time had been accepting many students that would not have been accepted elsewhere. It could be that Marshall's letters of recommendation gave some insight into somebody whose grades inadequately reflected his true potential.

Many of the current graduate students in the department had entered as World War II veterans. Marshall had been exempted from the war because of his rheumatic fever condition. Nonveterans didn't mix much with the veterans, many of whom had families and were close to finishing. Two of Marshall's closest friends at the time, Conrad Wagner and Raymond Holton, also had wives, while Marshall did not.[1]

Wagner had arrived at Michigan in January, a year earlier than Marshall. On his first plane trip ever, Wagner flew from New York City to a small airport in Rural Run, Michigan. Ann Arbor lacked an airport, so Wagner endured a ride of over 20 miles to reach the then frozen city. He eventually met Marshall for the first time in a lab on the ground floor of the West Medical Building on the main campus. There, graduate students including the newly arrived Marshall had assigned desks and spaces in which to work. Wagner found Marshall to be a "very charming, sweet guy. And he ... was ... interested in everybody. ... We hit it off right away."[2]

Built in 1902, the West Medical Building held both the research labs and classes for the biochemistry program. Facing the central campus, diagonal pathways connected buildings across a rectangular shaped central quadrangle. When Marshall crossed it with Wagner, it took Marshall 30 to 40 minutes, because he stopped to talk with everyone he knew. Wagner regarded Marshall as a thoughtful, caring person.

In the summer of 1952, Wagner and Marshall, along with other students from the department, took medical physiology. Medical students normally took the course during the year, but those who failed had to repeat in the summer. Therefore, the department of physiology offered medical students a summer remedial course, and the large number of chemistry and biochemistry students joined them. The accelerated course met five times a week and consisted of two hours of morning lecture and a lab spread out over the entire afternoon. Every Friday, Marshall and the other students turned in a lab report.

Marshall and Wagner worked together as lab partners in a building without air conditioning, a typical situation in the early 1950s. One set of experiments involved sacrificing a large turtle, dissecting out its heart, and studying how drugs affected the heart's contractions. Going through that course in the heat of the Ann Arbor summer felt like going through a battle. Lab partners bonded over the experience and became friends for life. In fact, Marshall and Wagner both ended up with the same mentor.

The two men had to write up the lab notes together, because neither could go at it alone. Marshall would join Wagner and his wife in their basement apartment on Thursday night to get the reports ready. Often, the three friends would go to dinner together. Then Marshall and Wagner would go back to the lab.

In addition to physiological chemistry, the graduate students faced four courses in physical chemistry, a more difficult subject for most. On his first exam, Wagner got a 48 and thought he failed. He later learned that was the class average. Two or three courses in organic chemistry added to their workload. Marshall did not want to spend time on all the classwork, preferring instead the challenges and solitude of lab research. He took some courses but not others, studied on his own, and passed all the finals. He had little trouble maintaining the minimum grade point average of B.

Marshall, despite skipping some coursework, managed to keep his grades up. However, they were not high enough to avoid the dreaded preliminary exams. Fortunately, Wagner's higher grades allowed him to be exempted from taking the exams, a prospect that terrified him. Marshall had to take the exams because he had skipped some of the courses. Failing the preliminary exam meant likely dismissal from the PhD program.

Raymond Holton remembers Marshall as "studious, quiet, pleasant, and ... very committed to doing well in his academic program."[1] Taking the preliminary exams required to continue in the program, Marshall impressed Holton with his ability to study intensely and write at greater length. "But," recalled Holton, "I did not see him as a brilliant scientist. Obviously I was a poor judge of intellect!"[1] Perhaps not, for many people underestimated Marshall over the course of his lifetime.

The university did not provide dormitories for most graduate students and those that had them faced restrictions on behaviors such as drinking beer. In addition, a housing shortage existed at that time in Ann Arbor. Marshall, like the others, grabbed the first available apartment. Year after year, students might switch apartments and roommates.

Marshall may have been the most eligible bachelor on the entire campus. His charm, good looks, height, dark wavy hair, and slight southern accent made him very appealing. As a teaching assistant, Marshall taught biochemistry labs for dental students, physical education majors, student nurses, and dental hygienists. As part of their course of study, dental hygienists, who were all women, needed volunteers to have their teeth cleaned. Hygienists would come over and try to sign Marshall up. So many hygienists wanted him that they stood in line outside the door to his lab. Marshall could never say no. As a result, Marshall had numerous girlfriends and very clean teeth.

Every Saturday from 10 a.m. to noon, Marshall and the other graduate students together with faculty attended seminar. Students read published papers and then presented their findings to the assembled department. One of the few women in the department came from the deep South, and Wagner thought he heard her once present on "bald rice." It took some time before he and Marshall realized that through her southern accent she really meant "boiled rice."

Wagner thought the quality of Marshall's seminar presentations exceeded those of the faculty. Marshall's enthusiasm, which he retained all his life, bubbled out in the way he spoke. Marshall, Wagner remembers, carried that enthusiasm into everything that he did. In 1953, Marshall selected for discussion a recent paper by Frederick Sanger on the sequence of amino acids, the building blocks of proteins, for the protein insulin. Sanger had begun publishing on the structure of insulin more than eight years earlier, but none of the courses at Michigan had mentioned it. The aging faculty in the biochemistry department had fallen behind the times. Marshall had not. Marshall intuitively recognized the importance of work that won Sanger a Nobel Prize five years later.

Marshall began as an assistant in the department and became a teaching fellow in September 1954. Marshall had some advantages over other graduate students in the department. Wagner, for example, remained unaware of how to use radioactivity for biochemical studies. Marshall knew about radioactivity from his work in the Nutrition Laboratory in Florida. Wagner later learned about radioactivity from a new faculty member who brought with him both experience and a Geiger counter to measure radioactivity.

Another relatively new faculty member, James Felter Hogg, a slow-talking Texan, brought the bloom of youth to the aging department faculty. Hogg had previously lived in New York. During World War II, Hogg experimented with how to produce enough penicillin to treat wounded soldiers. As a faculty member, Hogg had begun at Michigan only a few years before Marshall came. Hogg became an instructor for $3,600 annually. Hogg, who did not like to work late, contributed little to the research of the department. (By the time he retired, Hogg had published a paltry 14 or so scientific papers, in an era when 50 to 100 counted as average.)

Marshall and Wagner also shared a research lab together. Marshall knew that Wagner had chosen Hogg to be his advisor. Marshall had gotten to know Hogg, who had a warm and helpful personality. Now that Marshall had finished his courses and passed his oral exams, he also decided to choose Hogg as his thesis advisor. So Marshall went to the department chair, Lewis, to secure permission.

Shortly after, a crestfallen Marshall returned. Lewis had assumed Marshall wanted to work with him. Lewis wielded a great deal of influence in the field of biochemistry, knew every department chairman in the country, and ran an important placement service for graduate students. Marshall did not want to offend Lewis but did not know what to do. He feared the worst once Lewis learned the truth. Truthfully, Lewis's work on nutritional biochemistry did not appeal to Marshall who longed for a more up-to-date project on which to work. However, a week after meeting with Marshall, Lewis suffered a stroke while lecturing to medical students and never recovered.

Marshal, freed from his predicament, then selected Hogg to advise him. However, Hogg's limited research experience in biochemistry, not surprisingly, caused Marshall to struggle for a while with the research problem that Hogg had given him. Despite working hard on the problem, Marshall made little progress, as the problem proved intractable. This created a serious issue for Marshall: no successfully completed research, no PhD degree. The consolation prize would be another master's degree or possibly no degree at all.

Showing signs of his future experimental skills, Marshall on his own devised a new research problem that would garner his PhD. Using a type of cancer cell, Marshall investigated how one sugar blocked the cancer cell from using another sugar. The problem was a potentially interesting one because scientists already knew that cancer cells converted sugars into energy very inefficiently. Recalls Wagner, "I think Marshall's great ability was his imagination. ... He didn't have good hands in the lab but ... he got his experiments done well. ... Marshall would repeat things over and over again, and all the experiments were done carefully."[2]

Hogg liked to talk. Every Friday afternoon around four o'clock, Wagner would meet with him and together they would review the lab notes for the week. But Hogg could talk forever. Wagner wanted to get home to his young bride. Since Marshall remained single, Wagner would ask him to knock on the door after an hour to interrupt the meeting. As a result, it was Marshall who frequently ended up talking with Hogg for an hour or more on Friday nights.

With Lewis no longer able to function as the department chair, Halvor N. Christiansen came in to replace him. One day, Wagner, covered with a lab coat, sat on a lab stool while Marshall cut his hair. The two took turns cutting each other's hair to save money. Newly appointed, Christiansen burst into the room as part of his tour to see what went on in the department. Both Marshall and Wagner felt embarrassed as did Christiansen, who apologized and said, "I'll see you later," as he beat a hasty retreat down the hall.

Christiansen recruited new faculty including Minor J. Coon, who eventually met Marshall. "I had enough conversations with him," said Coon, "to immediately spot him as somebody who was very bright and exceptionally hard working. I was coming in at night myself sometimes, and he was just so enamored with doing research that one could predict that he would do well. But there's an enormous amount of luck with what happens to people."[3]

Coon characterized Christiansen as "demanding." "I think he ... felt that it was his responsibility to turn the department around and I think ... if he felt that some of the existing faculty were not going to be part of his future plan, he was quite honest with them about it."[3] Coon recalls that outside of Ann Arbor, hardly anyone knew the faculty of the department. The department changes made by Christiansen had relatively little effect on Marshall. He was well along in his thesis work by now. They did, however, affect Hogg, who departed for Queens College in New York soon after Marshall graduated.

Coon remembers that Marshall had many ideas and wanted to move ahead rapidly. But it was Hogg who insisted that all experiments be done repeatedly, although Coon thought sometimes excessively. He recalls, "It may have been a helpful message to Marshall that science requires many things, but among others, being absolutely sure of our results by repeated experimentation. So I would say that they were a very good pair, very different in personalities, but it turned out to be quite a good choice for Marshall."[3]

While Wagner ran experiments in the lab, his wife, Jane, worked for the phone company. One day, a coworker mentioned she needed to cut off a student's phone service because he hadn't paid his bill. Jane found out it was Marshall, who—wrapped up in his work—frequently forgot to cash his checks, which totaled about $1,200 a year. Jane helped Marshall straighten out his account and maintain his phone service.

By the time he finished, Marshall had experimented with biochemical techniques and had accumulated publishable data. And so in 1957, the University of Michigan granted Marshall Warren Nirenberg his PhD. Hogg advised him to hasten to the National Institutes of Health, a large research institution operated by the federal government, in Bethesda, Maryland. There, Marshall could benefit by improving his use of biochemical methods. Hogg had also recently met with the NIH's DeWitt Stetten Jr., who, Hogg believed, wanted Marshall as a potential postdoctoral applicant.

Marshall took Hogg's advice and, with a modest fellowship from the American Cancer Society that would pay $7,800 for two years, he left Ann Arbor. His health had prospered. He had survived both the cold of the harsh Michigan winters and the heat from sweating over experiments that too often failed to work. He had recast himself from observant zoologist to somewhat robust biochemist. Based on his placid years as a student and young scientist, he could hardly imagine that a life of scientific adventure awaited him.

5 No "Holes" Barred

In 1956, Marshall's second year of graduate school in the biochemistry department at the University of Michigan in Ann Arbor, Francis Crick appeared. Crick was on a tour and becoming a scientific icon. It was just three short years since Crick and Jim Watson had published their ground-breaking, epochal paper on the physical structure of DNA. Scientists believed that DNA controlled heredity by controlling the activities of cells. Watson and Crick showed that DNA had a chemical structure resembling a spiral staircase. At Michigan, Crick delivered a series of lectures in July, having first participated in a symposium on the chemical basis of heredity at Johns Hopkins University in Baltimore. Presumably, Marshall would have attended the lectures Crick presented at Michigan. For Crick, interspersed between visits to Baltimore and Ann Arbor, there was a stint as a visiting scientist at the National Institutes of Health and a lecture he gave in Madison, Wisconsin.[1]

Marshall and Crick were to cross paths many times again—as they would five years later, once Marshall announced his initial findings of a genetic code at an international meeting in Moscow. Over his lifetime, Marshall would give numerous interviews, jot down ideas and names in dozens of notebooks, and write about his discovery in scores of papers. Yet, with the exception of his meeting Crick in Moscow, Marshall failed to note any of his thoughts about Crick, or even mention Crick by name. This lack of acknowledgment probably reflected Marshall's later experiences with Crick and the personal gulf between the two men.

One scientist attending a dinner remembered Crick as "tall, thin, not as talkative as Sydney Brenner, but infinitely more talkative than Marshall Nirenberg. ... Bantering, you know, sparkling eyes with ladies. I think he enjoyed being flirtatious, for the sake of it, not because there was anything behind it at that stage. ... Entertaining ... he certainly talked about things of his past, you know, stories. He was a good storyteller. ... Because of who he was, people were listening more. That's the best way I can put it. He was interesting, of course."[2]

Marshall eschewed attention, preferring instead the solitude and excitement of lab work. While personable and friendly, he labored quietly, constantly, and intently. Marshall seemed by nature to favor solitude and independence. He had actually enjoyed the time when, recovering from rheumatic fever at age 10, he had spent an entire year mostly alone, unable to attend school. Then, Mel Shader had tutored Marshall in Mount Vernon, but the rest of the time Marshall spent reading. In Orlando, he roamed the swamps of his teenage years, for the most part, alone. At NIH, Marshall would initially lead a somewhat secretive life as he explored how cells make proteins.

Crick had the opposite personality. He adored attention and seemed to have grown up in a much more social world. His visit to the University of Michigan, for example, capped a five-month odyssey around the globe. He attended meetings, visited scientists, and discussed the discovery he made jointly with Jim Watson on the structure of DNA. Watson, who shared a Nobel Prize with Crick for the groundbreaking work, once wrote of him, "I have never seen Francis Crick in a modest mood."[3] François Jacob, another Nobel Laureate, recalled a talk that Crick gave in Paris: "He talked incessantly. With evident pleasure and volubly, as if he was afraid he would not have enough time to get everything out. Going over his demonstration again to be sure it was understood. Breaking up his sentences with loud laughter. Setting off again with renewed vigor at a speed I often had trouble keeping up with. A formidable intellectual machine."[4]

George Gamow Joins Forces with Crick and Watson

In July 1953, eight years before Marshall would reveal his stunning findings in Moscow, Crick and Watson received a letter from the astronomer George Gamow. He expressed an interest in the problem of the genetic code (the term scientists used for the alphabet of life). Made up of just four letters that stood for specific chemical units, information encoded into the structure of DNA made it the focus of cells. How could the simple spiral staircase structure of DNA enable it to direct the myriad activities of cells? Somehow, DNA held the instructions for life. But how, and in what form? The answers to these questions required scientists to translate the structure of DNA into some intelligible language.

Gamow had been trained as a theoretical physicist. Somehow, amid his pursuits of things universal in astronomy, Gamow felt a kinship with

Watson and Crick. Perhaps it was due to the decisive role physics had played in the DNA discovery. In his letter, Gamow referred to Watson and Crick's recent paper on DNA suggesting that "the precise sequence of the bases[letters] is the code which carries the genetical information."[5]

Gamow had also seen a recent paper that for the first time showed the precise order in which amino acids became strung together in a chain to build a protein. The protein structure belonged to insulin.[6] Scientists would soon realize that each protein is composed of a unique order of amino acids in a chain. The amino acids are bonded one to the next in each chain.

Gamow combined the ideas of both papers into a scheme by which the physical structure of DNA itself formed a pattern on which amino acids could be assembled directly into protein. In Gamow's scheme, DNA acted directly without an intermediate. And so Gamow's attention swung from the infinite expanse of the heavens to the molecular minutiae of genetics.

A Unique Club Forms

Gamow's theory led to the establishment of the so-called RNA Tie Club, which was initiated at the Woods Hole Oceanographic Institution in Massachusetts. Having succeeded with DNA, Watson wanted Crick and Gamow to now attend to RNA. Building blocks denoted with the letters A, T, G, and C help build large biological structures such as DNA. RNA, another large biological structure, is built the same way with U's substituting for T. Each structure runs as a chain. DNA has two chains and resembles a spiral staircase. RNA has just one chain. In 1957, both seemed composed of seemingly random combinations of these lettered building blocks. Both DNA and RNA figured strongly in the chemical basis of heredity. Exactly how remained unknown. Unlike DNA, confined to the cell's nucleus, RNA gallivants throughout cells in a variety of sizes. In 1952, Watson had predicted that DNA might not function directly to make protein but instead would need an intermediate, and he saw that RNA might be that intermediate. A year later, Watson began an as yet unsuccessful search for the structure of RNA. As Matt Ridley, a Crick biographer, writes: "While driving along a California freeway one day in the spring, Watson and the chemist Leslie Orgel ... conceived the idea of a club for people interested in RNA, an idea Gamow ... quickly ... took over. The "RNA Tie Club" was to have 20 members, each one with a necktie adorned with a squiggly RNA and a unique tie pin bearing the abbreviation for one of the 20 amino acids commonly found in proteins."[7]

Subsequently, Crick, Watson, and Gamow formed the RNA Tie Club. They initially planned to probe the role of RNA in protein synthesis. But they got increasingly drawn into how a genetic code might work. Orgel and Gamow worked on the design of the tie, which Watson then took to a Los Angeles haberdasher. The shop tailor made the ties for $4 apiece. Each of the 20 amino acid designs signified a member of the RNA Tie Club. Each member also received a golden tiepin with the abbreviation for that amino acid.

As the new members of the RNA Tie Club assembled together, Marshall slogged through his classes. He had emerged from the probation of his first year at the University of Michigan. He would graduate with a less than stellar academic record, with his advisor James Hogg sending him off to NIH "to develop his technical abilities."[8] Meanwhile, the membership of the RNA Tie Club would encompass mature scientists of such world renown that six would eventually carry the title Nobel Laureate—James Watson (biologist), Francis Crick (biologist), Sydney Brenner (biologist), Max Delbrück (physicist), Richard Feynman (physicist), and Melvin Calvin (biologist). The membership would also include Alexander Rich (biochemist), Paul Doty (physical chemist), Robert Ledley (mathematical biophysicist), Marynas Ycas (biochemist), Robley Williams (electron mictroscopist), Alexander Douce (biochemist), Norman Simmons (biochemist), Edward Teller (physicist), Erwin Chargaff (biochemist), Nicholas Metropolis (physicist and mathematician), Gunther Stent (physical chemist), and Harold Gordon (biologist).

An "old boys' network" helped the membership coalesce. Gamow induced Feynman, Metropolis, and Teller, and likely, Ycas, Ledley, and Rich to join. Crick invited Orgel and Brenner. Watson likely urged Doty, Dounce, Chargaff, and Delbrück to join. Exactly how others became members is unclear. Delbrück, then at the California Institute of Technology, might have invited Calvin, Simmons, Williams, and Stent, all of whom occupied positions in California institutions. By comparison, Marshall, a mere graduate student at the time and unknown, lacked any achievement, stature, and recognition from his peers.

Delbrück may have also influenced the club's development. He led the so-called phage group, a possible model for the RNA Tie Club. (Phage is a shortening of "bacteriophage," which are viruses that infect bacteria.) The phage group brought together like-minded scientists with a common goal of understanding how these viruses worked. The viruses served as experimental model organisms.

The phage group operated informally and encouraged others to join. Beginning in 1945, Delbrück and others at Cold Spring Harbor Laboratory taught young scientists the fundamentals of phage biology. The idea was to bring a physics and mathematical approach to biological research. Marshall himself would later take advantage of a phage course at Cold Spring Harbor.[9]

Remembering Max Delbrück, Seymour Benzer, physicist turned biologist and geneticist, recounted:

Delbrück could be extremely opinionated. He often had rather fixed ideas. The most extreme example I can think of is one in the later years when I was here. One of my students was interested in the biological clock; and he had shown that you could make mutations that changed the biological clock in ... [fruit flies]. And he was telling this to Max, and Max said, "No, that's impossible." And then I said, "But Max, he's already done it." And Max said, "No, that's impossible." That was not a completely unusual kind of event. ... It was often a very great source of stimulation that Delbrück would tell you something's impossible. You'd go ahead just to prove him wrong. The fact was, he had been wrong scientifically on many occasions. But as Jim Watson once said, "The difference between Max Delbrück and this other guy is that both have been very often wrong. But when Max is wrong, it's usually for an interesting reason."[10]

Whatever its origins, the RNA Tie Club differed significantly from the phage group. Whereas the phage group welcomed new members, the RNA Tie Club kept others such as Marshall out. Membership remained restricted to just the initial, select 20. The phage group offered instruction and shared knowledge; the RNA Tie Group remained reticent about its theories on the code. Apart in its private world, the RNA Tie Club acted in a manner distinct from the usual scientific process.

The bedrock of science rests on shared knowledge. In hallways, at meetings, in emails or on the phone, scientists freely exchange data and ideas. For example, Crick and Watson both attended a 1956 meeting on the chemical basis of heredity and presented on the structure of DNA and of RNA, respectively. However, neither man contributed in the formal discussions, at least, about their ongoing code work. Unlike other scientists, members of the RNA Tie Club nurtured their ideas in private. But that did not hold back Crick from tramping all over the globe. He queried scientists for their as-yet-unpublished data to support or refute his theories. Crick would then share the results by publishing them.

Yet the inner machinations of the RNA Tie Club remained insular. So much so that even graduate students at the California Institute of Technology at the time, when both Delbrück and Watson held forth on the faculty, never heard a word about it. Even today says one, "I don't know anything about the RNA Tie Club except what you can read about it in various books."[11]

Lubricated with alcohol and cigars, meetings of the RNA Tie Club tended to be friendly, cordial affairs. Men bonded together, exchanged ideas about a possible genetic code, and formed new friendships. Exchanges of letters and preprints of articles sallied back and forth between the meetings held twice yearly. But not all members engaged equally in the process. Crick became by force of personality the major figure of the RNA Tie Club. He extended his role to encompass laboratories all over the world.

The RNA Tie Club's theoretical approach to the code balanced on the shoulders of Crick and Watson and their prior success with DNA. The pair had successfully used theory to get the chemical structure of DNA. They couldn't see the structure directly. It lay beyond the vision of the most powerful microscopes of the era. They could only infer the structure from theoretical calculations and odd-looking dotted patterns gathered with X-rays. As closeted theorists, however, they found themselves vitally dependent on laboratory experimentalists. The experimentalists gathered the actual data and indirect evidence of the structure of DNA. How Watson and Crick acted to uncover the structure of DNA would later reverberate with Marshall in the race to discover the genetic code.

The laboratory experimentalists in the study of DNA included Rosalind Franklin and Maurice Wilkins. Wrote historian Robert Olby, "As we have learned from Watson's account in [his book] *The Double Helix,* he felt some embarrassment regarding the manner in which he and Crick gained access to [Rosalind] Franklin's data. Crick, it seems, was not free from some embarrassment either."[12] (Without consulting Franklin, Wilkins had shared her groundbreaking work in X-ray diffraction of DNA with Watson and Crick.)

Maurice Wilkins whose X-ray analyses of DNA also helped Watson and Crick formulate their winning structure, engaged repeatedly with Crick on the question of proper acknowledgment of his own contributions.[12] Wilkins eventually became a co-recipient with Watson and Crick of the Nobel Prize. Similarly, Watson and Crick may have also slighted Erwin Chargaff, who experimentally discovered that the ratios of the letter bases G:C and A:T in DNA both equaled one. Chargaff's observation was critical to the idea of pairing the two strands making up DNA. Watson and Crick relegated it to a mere reference in their paper on the spiral staircase structure.[13]

Marshall would later also come to feel the displeasure of Watson and Crick, as well. As far as is known, for example, neither man in their own published papers acknowledged Marshall and Heinrich Matthaei's later discovery of an RNA intermediate for DNA. This RNA is a copy of a portion of DNA and plays a central role in how proteins get made. Even in an exhaustive biography in which Crick is quoted at length, no such acknowledgment appears.[14]

Perhaps Crick best expressed the rationale for favoring Brenner's and Watson's separate but later discoveries of messenger RNA in the following words: "The only thing one can be thankful for is that it wasn't all done by someone, as it were, outside the *magic circle* [emphasis added], because we would all have looked so silly. As it was, nobody realized just how silly we were."[14] In his comment about looking "silly," Crick likely alluded to the embarrassment that would have been felt had someone else outside the RNA Tie Club discovered messenger RNA. Thus, the RNA Tie Club had to overlook Marshall and Matthaei's earlier discovery. Neither Marshall nor Matthaei would ever become part of the "magic circle." They could not be acknowledged and therefore had to be ignored.

Only two years removed from graduate school, unknown and unappreciated, Marshall had quite a different view. Unlike Crick, he had yet to cause a sensation in science. Few thought he ever would. How did he feel? In his private notebook, he wrote:

Most people who have [achieved] are committed to retain [their status,], and thus they have a stake in either maintaining the status quo or furthering their own way of thinking. The ones who don't have [any achievement yet] are uncommitted, and possibly their great asset is their lack of committedness although most do not realize it. It is possible, however, to have [achieved] and yet not be committed—only if one does not care about retaining [one's status]—if one can freely accept the loss."[15]

Theory versus Experimentation

Watson and Crick used the same "template" for solving the problem of the genetic code as they had for the structure of DNA. If theory worked once, theory would work again. As a result, the membership of the inner circle of the RNA Tie Club reflected their view. Gamow's background as a theorist also helped entice other theorists like Teller, Feynman, and Metropolis. Almost half the membership, and certainly the most active club members, evinced a theoretical outlook to the coding problem. The club members would become so wedded to a theoretical approach to the code that they would be unable to divorce themselves from it.

Eventually, on a global stage, the closeted theoretical approach of the RNA Tie Club would come up against the laboratory-based experimental approach of Marshall and others. The stakes for all involved would be enormous. Whoever published substantive data first, and gained priority, would be in line for at least a nomination for the Nobel Prize, the holy grail of scientific achievement. Intelligent, ambitious, and often very aggressive, the scientific elite of the RNA Tie Club might have proven an even more formidable obstacle to Marshall had they fully recognized the limits of theory.

Crick and Watson's proposed spiral staircase structure for DNA depended on pairing of letters such as A to T and G to C. Just three years later, Crick already envisioned how RNA might pair with DNA. He suggested that chains built chemically with a single letter found in natural DNA, like perhaps AAAAAAAAAAAAAA, could be tested with a similar chain-like UUUUUUUUUUUUUU. Each chemical chain could then be modified somewhere along the chain to see how the change might affect pairing.[16]

Marshall, not Crick, would later independently recognize that UUUUUUUUUUUUUU could be used for far more than just pairing of DNA to RNA: it could break open the logjam of ideas on how the genetic code worked. The key would be to make extracts of cells that could still make new protein in a test tube. UUUUUUUUUUUUUU might work as an unnatural messenger RNA to direct the production of a protein. Marshall would need to adjust the extract conditions until the extracts proved reliable, optimal, and productive.[17] If Crick had similarly recognized that possibility, he—not Marshall—might have won the Nobel Prize for the discovery of the genetic code.

Marshall realized that as a newcomer to this field of biology, he was at a considerable disadvantage. He drove himself incessantly. "You could get much more done in one day," Marshall exhorted himself. "Be more efficient and work harder. [The] key: [you] should be able to work efficiently even if you feel tired."[17] Eventually, Marshall would use UUUUUUUUUUUUUU to unlock how the genetic code worked. Crick and Watson were somewhat blindsided by their prior success with theory. As a result, they were unable to foresee fully the experimental value of UUUUUUUUUUUUUU.

As a member of the RNA Tie Club, Gamow used a simple form of combinatorial mathematics to suggest how a letter code could direct the assemblage of protein. Gamow suggested that each three letters of DNA directed one amino acid building block into its correct position in the chain that made a protein. Gamow had simply concluded that if the code for one amino acid building block consisted of one letter in the DNA structure, then only four amino acids could be encoded. The reason? Only four letters make up DNA. That would leave no possible letter combinations for the other 16 amino acids. Clearly, a one-nucleotide code would not work. Similarly, neither would a two-letter code, which would account for only 16 (4 × 4) letter combinations. So the *minimal* number of letters in the code, he reasoned, had to be 3 (4 × 4 × 4), which would give 64 possible combinations. For Gamow, who had used complex, advanced mathematics to theorize how the universe began, this was basically child's play. In fact, simple combinatorial mathematics like this is taught in third and fourth grade elementary school classes.[18]

Such theoretical calculations said little about the exact structure of the code or how it worked. It did not *prove* that three letters specified each one of the twenty possible amino acids. It merely suggested a possibility. Science demands rigorous proof, not theoretical speculation. Even if each possible three-letter code word directed one of each of the 20 amino acids into protein that still left 44 combinations unaccounted for. Did some or all amino acids use two or more three-letter combinations? Did all the amino acids respond to a three-letter code word or did some respond to a four-, five-, or six-letter code? Did all possible letter combinations have a coding function or were some of the 44 combinations nonfunctional? And, of course, there was the still unanswered key question: What were the exact letter combinations for each amino acid? These questions would be answered experimentally, unequivocally—not by the RNA Tie Club—but by Marshall. But Crick and members of the RNA Tie Club created such a strong tidal force publicly that Marshall must have felt he was swimming against a tide of opinion.

Gamow proposed that various combinations of letters making up the spiral staircase structure of DNA would form 20 "holes" (which Gamow called "rombs"). This was precisely the number needed to fit up to 20 amino acids into proteins.[19] The linear arrangement of the holes predicted that for any amino acid in a protein chain, the neighboring amino acid to the left and right would each be set. This fixation led to the concept of overlapping letters in which the three-letter combination for one amino acid affected the three-letter combination for each of its neighbors.

In 1955, Crick set out what was then known about a genetic code and what might yet be discovered about protein synthesis.[20] He posited a criticism of Gamow's overlapping code and suggested that data from known amino acid sequences in proteins could support his criticism. Brenner later expanded on Crick's suggestion in a published paper.[21] Crick noted that the *physical structure* of either DNA or RNA could not act directly as a pattern on which proteins could be made. But, he said, "each amino acid would be attached to an as-yet-unknown 'adaptor,' which would then align on the template." Yet the bewildering variety of possible codes led Crick to conclude, "In the comparative isolation of Cambridge I must confess that there are times when I have no stomach for decoding."[20]

Gamow's proposed code could be easily tested if one had the precise order of amino acids for various proteins found in nature. But the order of amino acids in proteins had only recently been realized. The British biochemist Frederick Sanger developed a method to do just that.[6] Prior to

Sanger's work, scientists assumed that proteins had no well-defined structure. Marshall had presented Sanger's paper in a department seminar while at the University of Michigan. But Marshall, then absorbed in his research on cancer cells, had done little else about Sanger's paper.

About the time that Marshall left Michigan for NIH, Brenner seized on published studies of the exact arrangement of amino acids in different proteins. Others had shown the exact order of amino acids in these different proteins. Brenner used these recent data to refute the idea of an overlapping code. Brenner analyzed the number of combinations of one amino acid with its neighbors. He found the actual combinations exceeded those theoretically possible in an overlapping code arrangement. So Brenner concluded an overlapping code was unlikely.

Brenner had assumed a genetic code word to be just three letters. However, if one had assumed a four-letter combination for each code word, then an overlapping code would be possible. Brenner did not address this possibility but adroitly assumed the number to be three.[21] Brenner may have chosen the simplest possibility. However, Brenner had little basis for assuming a three-letter code. In fact, some authors the following year did consider a code with four letters.[22]

Brenner may have picked up the idea of a three-letter code from a fellow club member, Alexander Dounce, who years before had proposed one. Perhaps not, for Brenner did not mention this earlier paper. But Marshall, who generously acknowledged and credited others, did not forget the origin of a three-letter genetic code. Marshall noted, Dounce "was far ahead of everybody else. ... He predicted that the code would be a ... [three-letter] ... code, and that ... RNA was the ... [pattern] ... for protein synthesis. But he buried this article in the proceedings of an Oak Ridge symposium. ... I was amazed when I finally read it. ... There was really very little known about ... [the production of] ... protein ... at the time.[9] Another member of the RNA Tie Club also acknowledged Dounce's idea of a three-letter code.[23]

Like Brenner, Crick also objected to Gamow's scheme because it failed to indicate in which direction, left or right, the chain of code letters would be read.[24] Without indicating direction, the arrangement of amino acids in each protein chain would be variable. But Sanger showed that the arrangement of amino acids in a chain for a particular protein was always the same, not random. Gamow also did not consider that insertion of each amino acid in a protein could be directed by more than one combination of letters. His scheme gave only 20 holes, one for each of the 20 possible amino acids. However, others pointed out that a total of 32 to 40 holes might exist, making multiple code words for one amino acid possible.[25] In any case,

Gamow's idea for the genetic code, like others proposed by members of the RNA Tie Club, would eventually be abandoned.

Marshall Comes to the Fore

By the time Marshall arrived in Bethesda, Maryland, to begin work at NIH in 1957, the RNA Tie Club had been laboring for four years. A meeting in nearby Baltimore on the chemical basis of heredity had concluded the year before. Marshall's arrival at NIH also came a year after the departure of Gamow from Washington, D.C., where Gamow had been on the faculty of George Washington University. (Gamow moved on to teach at the University of Colorado, where he would spend the rest of his career.) So the two men likely never crossed paths, at least not in Washington, D.C. But Marshall would unwittingly become the thorn in the path trod by Gamow and the others as they vigorously chased down how the letters in DNA encoded the precise patterns of amino acids seen in proteins.

Marshall's planned work was to focus on how sugars got into cancer cells. But once he came, Marshall almost immediately began to think about many of the same problems as those being hashed out by the RNA Tie Club. On December 31, 1957, for example, Marshall wondered whether DNA or RNA alone could transfer genetic characteristics into mice.[26] Marshall began planning such experiments, noting that they could be done in the nine weeks remaining to complete his other studies. Some 13 years earlier, DNA had been shown to alter genetic characteristics of bacteria. But scientists had been reluctant to accept these findings. How the arrangement of four letters in DNA could direct the exact arrangement of the up to 20 amino acids found in proteins remained a quandary.

In 1953, Watson and Crick had elucidated the DNA structure. Their discovery suggested a similarity between the linear structure of DNA and that of proteins.

The Discovery of sRNA

A year after arriving at NIH, Marshall remained focused on his postdoctoral experiments. But important discoveries related to the genetic code continued to pour forth. A research group at Massachusetts General Hospital identified a novel form of RNA they termed soluble or sRNA, for short.[27] This sRNA embodied Crick's proposed adaptor for amino acids. This adaptor would transport each amino acid to its correct position on a pattern provided by a hypothetical messenger RNA. A messenger RNA, imagined but not yet discovered, would be an intermediate between DNA and the production of protein. The messenger would be made of RNA and be a partial copy of DNA. As different adaptors lined up on the template, each with a specific amino acid, then the amino acids could be connected together with the specific arrangement each protein required. As the RNA template changed, so would the pattern for the protein it encoded.

Watson initially didn't know about the ongoing work in Massachusetts. On finding out, Watson expressed surprise that someone from outside the "magic circle" had found the proposed adaptor molecule. This exemplifies the struggle that occurs among scientists to be the first to make a discovery. Watson recalled being "a bit deflated and miffed at having the theoretical framework for our discovery foisted on us by an outsider —indeed by a molecular biologist—after we had revealed transfer RNA and correctly interpreted its significance!"[28] Watson would later advise up-and-coming students on the matter of scientific competition: "If it happens that someone else does win outright, better it be someone with whom you are on good terms than some unknown competitor whom you will find it hard not to at least initially detest."[29]

Marshall worked all day in the lab at NIH. In the quiet of the evening hours, he returned in his imagination and notebook jottings to the production of protein and the coding problem. Despite working long hours, Marshall remained a driven man. "Get busy!!!! Work. Stop cogitating," he directed to himself more than once.[30] Spurring himself to action had nothing to do with the RNA Tie Club, for at this stage Marshall probably was unaware of the group's existence. Even if he wasn't, it would have hardly mattered.

Crick summarized the evolution of the coding problem up to then as having passed through three phases: the vague, the optimistic, and now the confused. The confusion arose from the unexpectedly large variations found for the relative proportion of the four letters found for DNA from various sources. If a copy of DNA in the form of messenger RNA existed, the messenger RNA should show similar variations. But no one could find them.[22] What did it all mean?

Confusion would soon be erased by the actual discovery of messenger RNA—the postulated set of patterns that directed the arrangement of amino acids into proteins. Prior studies looked at ribosomal RNA—on which proteins are synthesized. Researchers did not yet realize that the ribosomal RNA contained only tiny amounts of the messenger RNA. The proportion of the four letters in the messenger RNA varied: the letter proportions of ribosomal RNA varied much less so. In 1959, Marshall would move to Gordon

Tomkins' group, where he would begin in earnest to study the genetic code. There, his imagination and thinking would blossom about how proteins get made and would lead him to the discovery of messenger RNA.

But in 1957 through part of 1959, Marshall remained unable to do any experiments on the code. His fellowship obligated him to work for others rather than alone as he wanted to do. So Marshall could only contemplate the possible studies he might carry out given the chance. His notebooks, however, show that he closely tracked the burgeoning numbers of scientific papers being published. The details of these experiments became the fodder that fed the stream of ideas pouring into his notebooks. Marshall became drawn to studies in which proteins changed as the DNA that gave rise to them changed.[31]

The work of François Jacob and Jacques Monod particularly fascinated Marshall. Monod's work showed that a protein could be induced to form by exposing bacterial cells to a chemical that stimulated the production of that specific protein.[32] Almost immediately, Marshall recognized that if he could isolate the messenger RNA for this protein, he might have a good experiment. He could analyze the order of both the letters in the messenger RNA and the order of amino acids in the protein. By linking the data from both, Marshall could possibly work out how many letters and which ones specified each of the amino acids.[33]

A valid idea but, at the time, an experiment impossible to do. Methods to analyze proteins had only recently been worked out.[6] How to study the arrangement of letters in DNA or RNA had not. Interestingly, the same person who developed the methods for proteins would later develop the methods for RNA and DNA. For his efforts, he would be separately awarded not one but two Nobel Prizes, one of only two people to have accomplished this in the same category. Yet, Marshall long persisted in believing that inducing the production of a protein held the key to understanding the genetic code. In this belief, his inexperience in this area of research betrayed him.

Members of the RNA Tie Club themselves recognized that neither mathematics nor theory offered the rigorous proof demanded by the genetic code and science, in general. Although the club thrived on theory, Crick, Brenner, and a few other members did seek experimental proof for a three-letter code. The most striking example appeared in a paper published as the year 1961 drew to a close.[34]

The paper, filled with terms such as "suggest," "likely," and "probably," indicate that this is as close as members of the RNA Tie Club got to explaining the genetic code. The authors used chemicals known as acridines to alter DNA. The basis of the changes had only been described a few months earlier.[35] The chemical acridines act by squeezing inside the spiral staircase of DNA. The physical distortions in the DNA introduce mistakes when the DNA is copied.[36] The authors were unable to see changes directly in DNA. They detected changes in the DNA indirectly based on how bacteriophage virus grew on different bacteria.

Chemical acridines were less than ideal for uncovering the genetic code. The authors could not be certain of how DNA changed. Crick and Brenner admitted as much, saying that the genetic code might consist of a combination of either three *or* six letters.

The study was a theoretical tour-de-force, but one that neither spelled out the exact number of letters nor what letter combinations were needed for each amino acid. Brenner himself admitted, "It was a real house of cards theory. You had to buy everything."[37] Crick agreed, saying, "It has yet to be shown by direct biochemical methods, as opposed to the indirect genetic evidence mentioned earlier, that the code is indeed a triplet code."[38]

The discovery of sRNA was made without knowledge of Crick's adaptor hypothesis. Neither would Marshall's discovery of the letter combinations making up the genetic code depend on the theories of the RNA Tie Club. Rather, Marshall would seek hard experimental evidence to define the genetic code. The discovery of sRNA would shortly help Marshall immeasurably. sRNA functioned as a key ingredient for the production of proteins. Whether or how the experimental data matched theory mattered less to Marshall than what his cell extracts revealed. However, to Crick, *how* experiments matched theory mattered a great deal. Experiments that validated his theories validated him.

In spite of the brainpower posed by the RNA Tie Club, its members did not ultimately fare well collectively in terms of winning the race to crack the genetic code. They would not be the first to propose the existence of messenger RNA or confirm its discovery. They had not discovered sRNA. They would be unable to prove the exact combinations of letters that spelled out the genetic code. They would not unequivocally show which letter combinations coded for which amino acid. Virtually the one finding on which the members could hang their collective hats would involve the letter combinations that signaled protein production to stop. In the summer of 1959, Marshall would start in earnest to make most of these key findings missed by the RNA Tie Club. In two years, in the race to the code, Marshall's rapid strides would draw him alongside the progress being made by members of the RNA Tie Club. Whether Marshall could surpass them would be spelled out over the next five years.

6   The Gates Open

Marshall felt elated in 1957 when he drove for the first time through the entrance to the National Institutes of Health (NIH) in Bethesda, Maryland. Leaving his apartment on East Huron Street in Ann Arbor for the final time, he guided his 4-door 1955 Chevy along Interstate Route 80, his car loaded with the meager belongings of a former graduate student. He had just bought the Chevy for $200 with a loan cosigned by his father.

As a newly minted PhD, Marshall found himself on the verge of fulfilling his dream of a career. Now thirty years old and somewhat older than many in his situation, he had high expectations as he embarked on postdoctoral training. Chafing under the standard training system that prevented him from becoming completely independent immediately after graduation, he hoped to transition quickly from dependency on a mentor to total research independence. In his pocket he carried fellowship support from the American Cancer Society that would pay the princely sum of about $3,900 annually for the next two years of training.[1]

As he went down Center Drive on the grounds of NIH that evening, Marshall looked up in amazement to see the lights on in many of the buildings. To Marshall this meant many NIH scientists worked late into the evening. He himself also preferred to work late when the day for most others was drawing to a close. He felt that the blaze of lights must surely be a good omen. Only later did Marshall realize that the lighted buildings held not late-working scientists but cleaning crews who came through once the laboratories closed at 5 p.m. A series of other disappointments awaited Marshall as well.

Marshall liked sugar. Not the type you savor but the type you study in cancer cells. This had been the basis of his research in Michigan. Now he eagerly awaited the opportunity at NIH to learn more about how sugars entered cancer cells and what happened to them once inside. His mentor at NIH, W. DeWitt Stetten Jr., it turned out, had other plans for Marshall.

Stetten did not immediately make this clear, however. Before Marshall arrived, Stetten had already left for the Woods Hole Oceanographic Institution in Massachusetts, where he spent much of each summer. Unfortunately, it had slipped Stetten's mind to share this news with Marshall. Brimming with enthusiasm and optimistic with plans, Marshall now unexpectedly found himself isolated and alone without a mentor—a second early disappointment for Marshall.

Marshall wanted to pursue several ideas about sugars. Glands in the body secrete hormones that exert powerful biological effects. How, Marshall wondered, might these hormones also affect cancer cells and their use of sugars? In the case of healthy cells, how would cancer-inducing agents alter their use of sugars?[2]

Such studies could yield important insights into the cancer process. The central role of sugar in cells could prove important. Sugars are altered within cells and, in the process, produce energy, which is stored in a special molecule. Cells use this molecule as a form of currency to "pay" for life activities that require, rather than generate, energy. Unlike healthy cells, cancer cells use sugar and produce energy in a wasteful way.

In an August 1957 letter to his former Michigan advisor James Hogg, Marshall wrote that he had found no effect of hormones on transport of sugar into cells. But the real gist of his letter to Hogg held a complaint about Stetten, who had admonished Nirenberg about doing any further independent work on sugars and cancer cells. This action Nirenberg summed up in one word: "unfair." Marshall noted:

[I had a] complete understanding that I would work on sugar transport and hormonal effects after leaving Ann Arbor. I worked [the] last 3–4 weeks to survey [the] field so that I would have promising leads to work on here. [I] told you that I wanted to present Stetten with experimental data—leads—so that he would give me independence to follow my own bent. This I have. No misunderstanding of this. I told you that even if he did not give his permission I would work on the problem in the evenings and weekends on my own time.[3]

Marshall as Taskmaster of Himself

Soon followed the first of a series of notebook entries in which Marshall seemingly berated himself about his work habits. "The holiday is over. Stop going in frustrated circles. Work in most efficient manner you can. Let nothing stop you. Get survey done!!"[4]

However, Marshall's success would ultimately rest not with sugars and cancer cells but with the chemical basis of heredity. DNA contains the

letters A, T, G, and C. RNA contains the same letters except for U in the place of T. The letters in both DNA and RNA stand for chemicals that when linked together compose the structures. In 1957, DNA and RNA seemed composed of seemingly random combinations of these letters. Both DNA and RNA figured strongly in the chemical basis of heredity. Exactly how remained unknown. A key question, therefore, in tracing Marshall's route to the Nobel Prize, is how did Marshall's thinking transition from cancer cells and sugars to the letters making up DNA and RNA?

Ignoring Stetten's directive to focus just on changes to sugars in normal cells, Marshall continued his studies after hours while seeking to stay below Stetten's radar. The sugar studies themselves suggested a connection to DNA and RNA. Marshall saw that cells use a few of the letters found in DNA to build derivatives. These derivatives help cells alter sugar and produce energy. Marshall envisioned sugars somehow becoming attached to the individual letters to make these derivatives.[5] Marshall saw other parallels, as well, between large sugar structures and DNA. Individual sugar molecules could be chemically hooked together to form long chains. To Marshall, this resembled the long stretches of letters in DNA and RNA.[6]

However, interacting with sugars is not the main function of the letters that make up DNA. DNA came to life with the publication in 1953 by James Watson and Francis Crick of its spiral staircase structure. Exactly how the chemical structure of DNA managed to run all the functions of a cell remained hidden in 1957. RNA too appeared to be essential to life. Marshall would eventually uncover the answer to the role of DNA and RNA in the form of coded instructions based on the arrangement of letters in DNA. In the process, Marshall would win a Nobel Prize.

In the 1940s, while Marshall still attended college, the biological activity of DNA, in particular, had been found capable of changing bacteria from one type to another. As the year 1958 began, Marshall's attention to the biology of DNA and RNA in his notebooks became more evident. Now Marshall envisioned a "marriage" of ideas between DNA and sugars. Marshall thought it possible to track how DNA and RNA could alter cells by checking how changes in DNA could alter how cells use sugar.[7]

Other ideas to track how DNA works quickly followed. For example, Marshall wondered what would happen if he incubated sperm with different DNAs? Would he see changes in genetic characteristics in the offspring? These seemingly DNA-altered sperm could be used to inseminate female mice, and the resulting litter could then be studied for changes. Interspersed with these ideas was the day-to-day gathering of data for sugar experiments that seemed increasingly routine. Marshall hoped these data would help win his research independence.

Yet Marshall retained cordial relationships with Stetten. "Stetten," Marshall remembered, "was a wonderful person—a wise, intelligent, literate individual, and extremely articulate. ... He had a wonderful sense of humor. Both he and his wife were extremely kind to me. ... They had parties and invited lots of people to their house, including visitors to the NIH. I met lots of people there."[1]

In the weeks that followed, Marshall flitted from one idea to another, from one experiment to another. "Use DNA-RNA to ... test the growth of different cancer cells, complete sugar experiments, get analyses ready for Stetten, prepare ... [DNA] ... ponder about a particular growth-promoting substance, and, of course, provide a measured dose of exaltation." "Get busy!!!! Work. Stop cogitating," he wrote to himself.[8]

Caught between Stetten's demands and his own strong impulses for independence, Marshall must have felt pressured and stressed. "Stop thinking at night. Do experiments." Still doing carbohydrate studies."[9] And again, "Overall philosophy. Must get up efforts to do ... work. Must therefore work hard and carefully. Don't do sloppy work."[10] And again, "Do clean work. No sense doing any experiment if it's done sloppily!!!" "Stop talking!!! and wasting time."[11] Clearly, Marshall, even at the outset and throughout his life, acted as a man driven to understand how life works.

He saw his overall philosophy as looking for biological problems, devising ways to solve them, and then profusely publishing the results. Yet, in a later notation, he decided he wanted to spend time doing groundbreaking work in other areas of biology that would lead to many more "misses" than "hits" and, consequently, fewer publications. Once good progress could be made on a problem, he would turn it over to someone else and move on to the next challenge.[12]

Marshall worked during the day in the lab. In the evening, he read and thought about DNA and RNA. He would devote at least half his time to looking for the next problem to solve. Contradicting what he had said before, he now reasoned that once he had a good bead on a problem, he would follow it tenaciously until completed. The key, Marshall decided, rested on being "extremely careful, meticulous and thorough until all loose ends of previous problems are tied up. Do not follow secondary problems yourself. ... This overall approach will primarily be nonproductive but will result in a small amount of highly original work."[12]

Marshall's concerns about his career melded with anxiety about getting a job. "Personal ambition should not mean anything to me," he wrote. "I cannot approach my potential by working alone. My motives for wanting to get a good job are therefore not primarily that I feel personal ambition.

This point up to now has been confused in my mind."[13] Although on further reflection Marshall decided to cross out these words, his initial impulse to write them shows concerns that weighed on his mind.

Marshall had more to fear than failure. His anxiety about a job reflected the difficulties his father had encountered in Orlando. As Marshall worried about his father, Harry worried about his son. "Apparently my father stopped in to see Dr. Stetten," Marshall related, "and wanted to know if he thought that I would be able to make a living as a biochemist, if I could get a job as a biochemist. He knew me pretty well. I was never interested in money basically, and he thought that I would do best maybe in an academic setting; so he simply wanted to reassure himself. I was very embarrassed when I found out about it, to tell you the truth, but it was important for him to know that I wouldn't be a total failure, at least."[1]

Marshall Expands His Knowledge Base

In 1958, Stetten assigned Marshall to work with William Jakoby, a brilliant scientist who had received his doctoral degree in microbiology from Yale University. Jakoby specialized in the study of enzymes—proteins that set in motion chemical reactions in cells but remain unchanged themselves. Marshall published three papers in prestigious science journals with Jakoby, one in the *Journal of Biological Chemistry*, one in the *Proceedings of the National Academy of Sciences*, and one in *Nature*. Yet, Marshall's laboratory skills did not particularly impress Jakoby.[14] Likely, Marshall's inexperience with enzymes contributed to Jakoby's impression.

Marshall realized that his education from Michigan was incomplete. His work with Jakoby enabled Marshall to learn more about the role of proteins in the life of a cell. He imagined this would be useful in his future work, whatever that turned out to be. Marshall's thinking later proved correct. The protein, polynucleotide phosphorylase, then being discovered, would prove critical to Marshall's own research. To make up deficiencies in his scientific knowledge, Marshall realized he might have to teach himself. In addition, he could take courses offered at NIH or other local institutions. In a few short years, Marshall would learn so quickly that he became a recognized leader of the chemical basis of heredity.

Unknown to Jakoby, Marshall focused as much free time as possible on the chemical basis of heredity. Even while Marshall worked with Jakoby, his mind obsessed over the latest advances concerning DNA, RNA, and proteins. He thought out experiments that he might someday conduct. His attention did not yet encompass the question of how information embedded in the structure of DNA got transferred into action within the cell. Instead, his first thoughts led to understanding how sperm form and mature, a problem Marshall considered "magnificent" and "untouched."[15]

About one month later, Marshall, not surprisingly, confessed confusion over his career. He felt he was traveling around aimlessly, looking in all directions for problems on which to work. Marshall so loved science that every problem, every paper, every new fact seemed to beg for his attention. Yet, he recognized the gulf between reading about a problem and actually working on it. Until he did a study, he had no way to know whether or not his solution might work.[16]

That a multitude of ideas continued to hound him incessantly actually boded well for Marshall's future. But the constant litany of ideas also provoked a sense of confusion that rendered him unable to separate major problems from minor ones. The barrage of potential ideas, though, continued unabated.

Cracking "Life's Code"

His first idea about the flow of information from DNA to proteins likely occurred in late November 1958. Marshall thought he could possibly trick a bacterial cell into releasing its DNA. He could then determine the order of letters that made up the DNA. Perhaps he could then relate the order of the letters in DNA to the arrangement of the building blocks that made up a protein. These building blocks were termed amino acids. Proteins were known to contain as many as 20 different types of amino acids arranged in linear chains. The term *genetic code* referred to how DNA spelled out the information that arranged amino acids in the correct order in each protein. Proteins differ both in the length of their chains and the arrangement of their amino acids. Marshall noted, "[I] would not have to get ... synthesis very far to break the coding problem. ... [I] could crack life's code!"[17]

While basically correct, a serious defect spoiled Marshall's plan. As Nobel Laureate Melvin Calvin once observed, anyone can come up with big problems of interest. The trick is to come up with a big problem that can actually be solved.[18] Marshall had identified a critical need to relate the structure of DNA to its content of information. But he had overlooked an important fact. His relative inexperience led him to think that he could find the order of letters in DNA. At the time, he could not. Methods to do so remained unknown.

However, other reported discoveries strongly stoked Marshall's interest. In France, François Jacob and Jacques Monod found a way to force DNA to express some instructions. They just had to present a bacterial cell with a bit of sugar. In particular, Marshall wondered if long chemical chains filled with negative charges might interfere if given to the bacteria after the sugar.[19]

By April 1959, Marshall found himself caught up in the outpouring of research papers on the functions of RNA and DNA. These studies, he predicted, would dominate biological research for the next 10 years. Little did Marshall know when he wrote those words that he would help make it happen. Marshall also read about a biological messenger, a postulated copy of DNA. He wondered if he figured out the order of letters in the messenger RNA, he might find for which protein it coded. He might also relate the messenger RNA to the portion of DNA from which it was copied. Yet, again, this idea would come to naught. Marshall had no way to determine the order of letters in DNA or RNA.[20] In two to five years, thought Marshall, details of how cells made proteins would be complete. "Probably 2 years," he noted.[21] It would actually take Marshall about seven years just to complete the work on how DNA directs the production of protein. Details of how protein synthesis works continue to emerge to this day.

Marshall thought that inducing a cell to form a new protein posed the best way to understand how protein got made. Giving sugar to a bacterial cell induced the cell to make a new protein. If a radioactive amino acid, one of the building blocks of protein was present, it would be chemically added into the new protein. The amount of radioactivity in the protein would then equate with the amount of new protein made.

Marshall figured he could also use virus to look for the hypothetical messenger RNA. To test this idea, he could infect bacteria with a virus. Once inside the bacterial cell, the virus would set its DNA to work. Marshall could possibly isolate the messenger RNA copied from the DNA. He could then determine the order of letters in the messenger RNA. He would also determine the order of amino acids in the new protein being made in response to the messenger RNA. The idea of correlating the order of letters and amino acids came ahead of its time.[22] Marshall would have had to invent methods to determine letter order in the messenger RNA and amino acid order in the protein. The invention would itself be a major undertaking. Marshall must have realized these limitations. He continued to work out these ideas on paper but not in his lab. He noted, "My main aim is not to crack … [how] … protein … [gets made] … but to have everything ready to study … [protein] … induction."[22]

A short time later, Marshall went back to ideas about producing protein in a test tube. The key, he decided, required evidence of *new* protein made. He would add supplements to the test tubes, "including the kitchen sink," but would keep controls to a minimum initially. "Include every dog-brained idea you get," he admonished himself. "One might work."[23]

Unsure of how to plan his career, Marshall sought advice from a post-doctoral fellow who had just worked with biochemist Feodor Lynen. Lynen would soon win the Nobel Prize for his work on cholesterol and metabolism. The fellow had asked Lynen for advice if he were just beginning in biochemistry and picking a problem to start a career. Lynen advised choosing a problem of great interest, one to get really excited about, and in which other people also expressed interest. Don't worry about competition, said Lynen, because even if someone else publishes first, you'll do it in a different way, and it will also be publishable. "So," said Marshall, "that's the philosophy that I used."[1] When Marshall later met Lynen and related this story to him, Lynen denied the story.

By then it was too late. Marshall had committed his time, energy, and resources to his new love of DNA, RNA, and protein. He would plunge into the flood of papers flowing from the publishing presses and dive into one study after another. But Marshall was also gambling with his career. If he failed on the project he was about to undertake, another job in research might be beyond his reach. Lynen might have trivialized the competition issue. But Marshall would soon face the white-hot heat of competition from three groups that could cause even the best of men to falter.

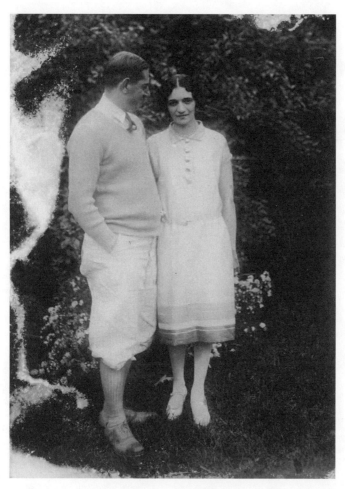

Plate 1
Harry Nirenberg and Minerva Bykowsky, Marshall's parents, around the
time of their engagement in 1924. (Courtesy of Beverly Geiger Bonnheim.)

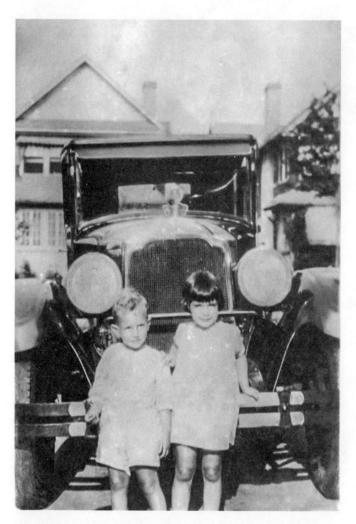

Plate 2
Marshall and his sister Joan in Brooklyn, New York. (Courtesy of Beverly Geiger Bonnheim.)

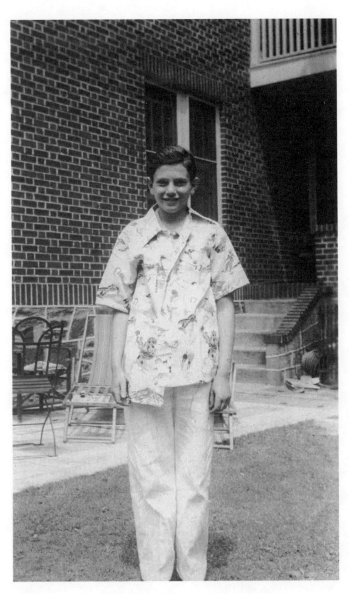

Plate 3
Ten-year-old Marshall recovering from rheumatic fever in Mount Vernon, New York. (Courtesy of Beverly Geiger Bonnheim.)

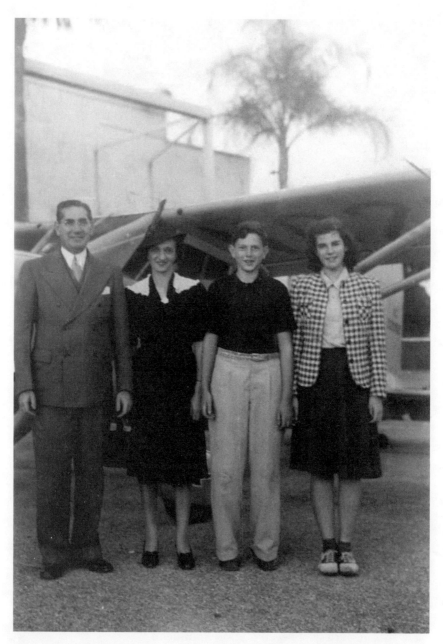

Plate 4
From left to right, Harry, Minerva, Marshall, and Joan around the time of their arrival in Orlando, Florida, in 1937. (Courtesy of Beverly Geiger Bonnheim.)

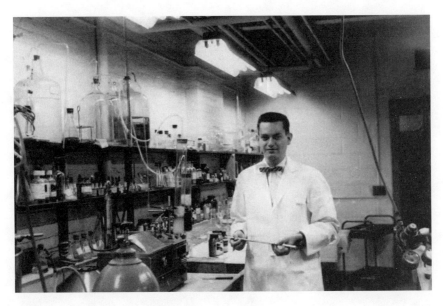

Plate 5
Marshall in his laboratory at NIH, circa 1960. (Courtesy of Beverly Geiger Bonnheim.)

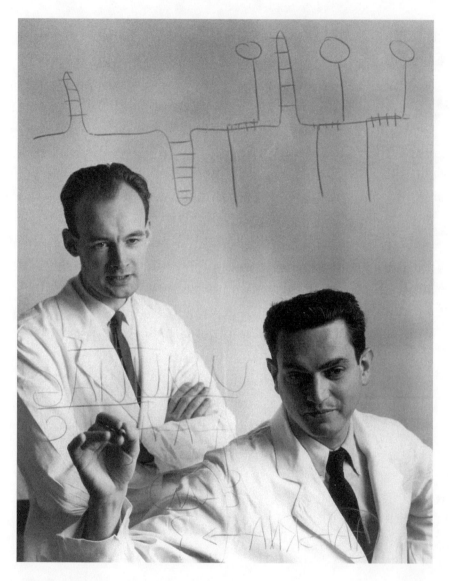

Plate 6
Marshall Nirenberg and Heinrich Matthaei, circa 1961. (Courtesy of the Stetten Museum of Medical Research, NIH.)

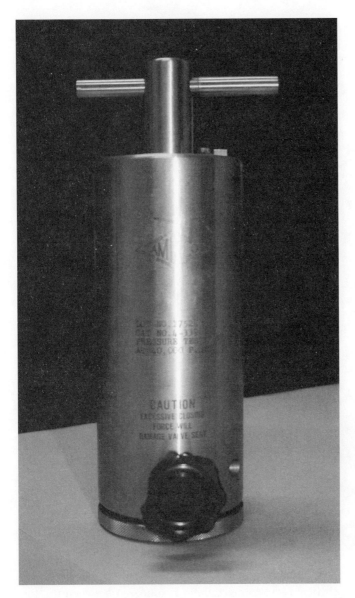

Plate 7
French press chrome cylinder, side elevation. Pressure cell used to prepare cell extracts. When the spigot at the base of the pressure cell is opened, the sudden drop in pressure as the cells, suspended in liquid, exit causes the cells to burst open. (Courtesy of the Stetten Museum of Medical Research, NIH; Hank Grasso, photographer.)

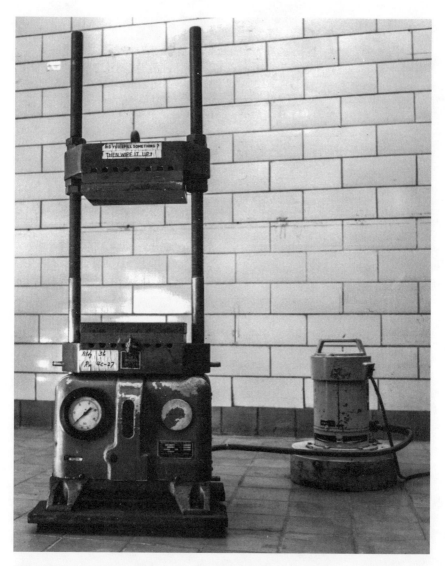

Plate 8
When the piston within the chrome cylinder is squeezed between the top and bottom surfaces, high pressures are generated within the cylinder. (Courtesy of the Stetten Museum of Medical Research, NIH.)

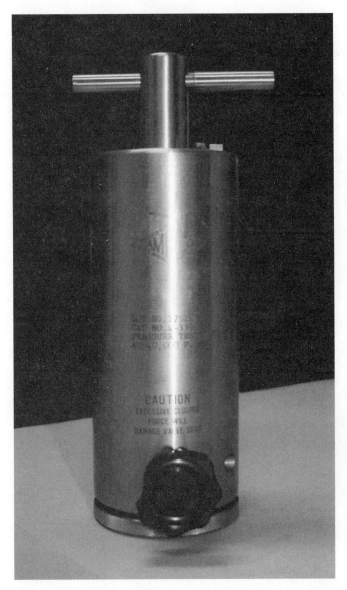

Plate 7

French press chrome cylinder, side elevation. Pressure cell used to prepare cell extracts. When the spigot at the base of the pressure cell is opened, the sudden drop in pressure as the cells, suspended in liquid, exit causes the cells to burst open. (Courtesy of the Stetten Museum of Medical Research, NIH; Hank Grasso, photographer.)

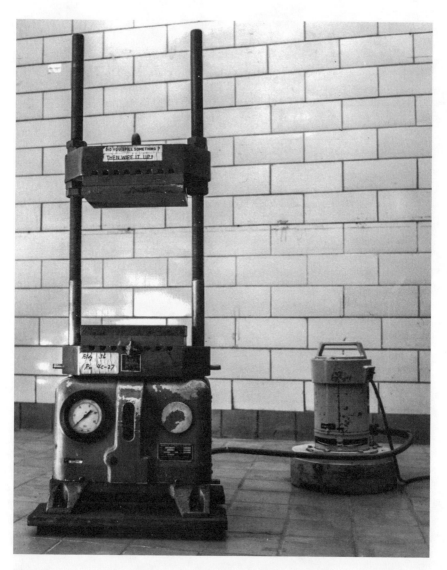

Plate 8
When the piston within the chrome cylinder is squeezed between the top
and bottom surfaces, high pressures are generated within the cylinder.
(Courtesy of the Stetten Museum of Medical Research, NIH.)

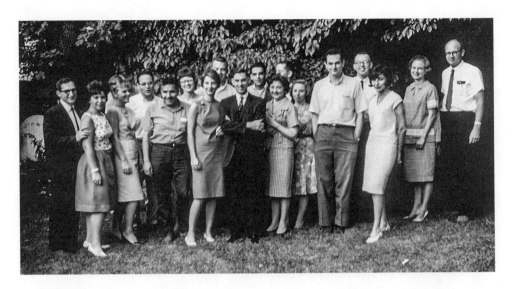

Plate 9

A photo used in a 1964 article by Marshall Nirenbrg. From left to right: Sid Petska, Joan Pestka, Margaret Clark, Tom Caskey (partially hidden), Dick Marshall, Taysir Janoui, Carol Rottman, Norma Zabriski Heaton, Fritz Rottman, Brian Clark, Philip Leder, Anna Shapiro, Joel Trupin, Kathryn Trupin, Marshall Nirenberg, Bill Groves, Perola Nirenberg, Bertie O'Neal, and Charles O'Neal. (Courtesy of the Stetten Museum of Medical Research, NIH.)

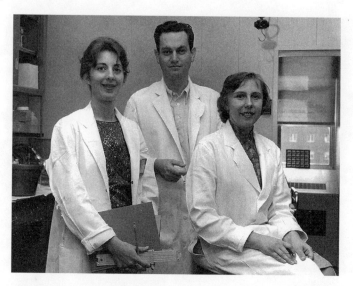

Plate 10

Marshall Nirenberg and his two devoted laboratory technicians, 1964. Theresa Caryk (right) worked with Marshall for 12 years. Norma Zabriski Heaton (left) stayed for almost 40 years. (Courtesy of the National Library of Medicine, Jerry Hecht Collection.)

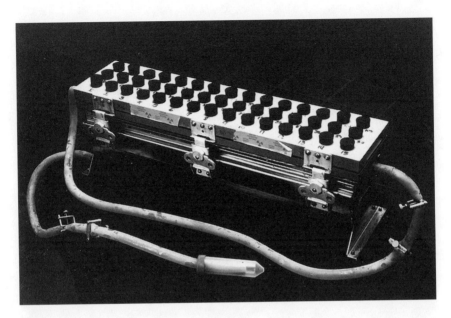

Plate 11

Invented by geneticist Philip Leder, the multi-plater is connected to a vacuum. The contents of each of 45 test tubes is poured separately onto a filter in each well. The rubber stoppers are reinserted and the vacuum pulls through the filter unreacted materials. Then each filter is removed with tweezers and placed in a vial for counting radioactivity. (Courtesy of the Stetten Museum of Medical Research, NIH.)

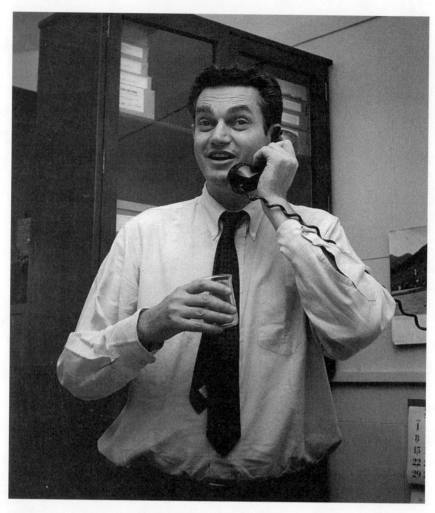

Plate 12
Marshall Nirenberg on telephone receiving congratulations for winning the
Nobel Prize. (Courtesy of the National Library of Medicine.)

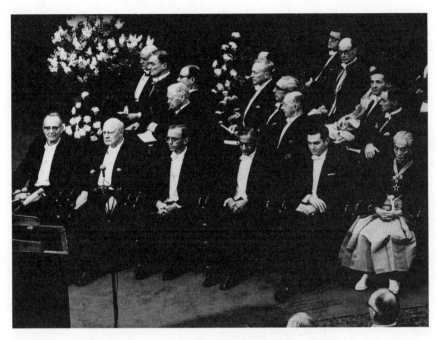

Plate 13
The Nobel Prize ceremony in 1968. Marshall is in the front row, second from the right. (Courtesy of Beverly Geiger Bonnheim.)

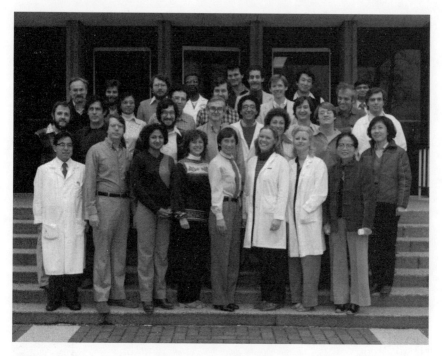

Plate 14

The members of a Nirenberg neurobiology group, circa 1977. From left to right: Saburo Ayukawa, Neil Busis, Satya Dandekar, Anne Schaffner, Mary Ellen Michel, unidentified, unidentified, Alice Ling, Angel de Blas, Ilan Spector, Katie Daruwalla, Matthew Daniels, Marshall Nirenberg, Michael Schneider, Celia Gazdar, Joseph Moskal, Kenneth Weeks, Maria Shih, Douglas Kligman, Paul Darveniza, David Trisler, Yitzhak Koch, Steven Sabol; Alan Peterkofsky, Fiorenzo Battaini, Michael Adler, unidentified, Zvi Vogel, William Strauss, Yoshiyuko Takahara, and Radharaman Ray. (Courtesy of National Institutes of Health, Office of NIH History; from the Branson Collection: Will and Ernie Branson, photographers.)

7   Revelations

In the summer of 1956, Marshall, in an effort that would eventually fail, wrestled with his assigned research for his PhD degree. Stress from the failure of his research added to his discomfort of working in university buildings that lacked air conditioning. It did not help that a heat wave enveloped the city of Ann Arbor. Eventually, Marshall on his own would redesign the study on sugar and cancer cells and graduate.

Meanwhile, halfway across the country in Baltimore, Maryland, an august group of scientists gathered to discuss how DNA, the genetic material, managed to direct the myriad activities of cells. Against a rising backdrop of addiction in the city spurred on by young whites experimenting with heroin, Nobel Laureates and lesser dignitaries, almost all white males, assembled at Johns Hopkins University to discuss the chemical basis of heredity.

Papers from this symposium would eventually engage Marshall's budding interest in a key question: how exactly did DNA work? Yet some of the "discoveries" mentioned in this meeting would later be proven wrong. Not realizing that would hinder Marshall's later research and that of others to understand the functions of DNA. The meeting presentations, published the year after Marshall left Michigan, would alter the direction of his interests, career, and life.

William David McElroy and H. Bentley Glass, the organizers of the Baltimore conference, both evoked a strong curiosity and a propitious sense of timing. Glass focused on the genetics of organisms that ranged from miniscule fruit flies to the admixture of genes between Negroes and American Indians. McElroy chased the abundant fireflies that flitted about the campus of Johns Hopkins University and, after he caught them, discovered how they managed to emit light.[1]

Several recent seminal discoveries drove this newfound interest in the chemistry of heredity. One was the central role that DNA might play. Oswald T. Avery and his associates had discovered that adding DNA from one organism could transform another.[2] Despite being highly regarded by his peers, Avery's claim that DNA and the genetic material were one and the same earned little respect. Researchers had already found only four different chemical blocks called nucleotides or bases (represented by the letters A, G, C, and T) in DNA. They also knew that proteins carry out the many activities of life. If DNA held the blueprint of life, how did that give rise to proteins? DNA had just four building blocks. But proteins had as many as 20 different ones. The set of building blocks in proteins are called amino acids. Particularly puzzling was how DNA with its four letters could arrange the as many as 20 different amino acids found in proteins. How could just four do the work of 20? It just didn't add up.

Answers to these questions would guide a better understanding of cell processes. Those processes depend to a large extent on the actions of proteins. So the recent progress made in knowledge of DNA and RNA fed hopes that similar progress could be made on protein production. The curiosity of scientists was piqued by the fact that DNA, RNA, and proteins could all be described as linear chains. Stretched out, each chain somehow seemed related to the others. But scientists remained in the dark about how this all worked.

Confirming DNA's Role in Protein Synthesis

A debate raged. Could DNA, in fact, direct the synthesis of proteins? Many scientists believed that, more likely, proteins somehow directed their own synthesis. Less than a decade after Avery's work, Alfred D. Hershey and Martha Chase at the Cold Spring Harbor Laboratory in Long Island, New York, confirmed the central role of DNA. They designed a kitchen-like experiment using a Waring Blendor. First, they exposed bacteria to a type of viral particle called a bacteriophage. They had grown the viral particle in a solution of radioactive materials. The DNA contained one type of radioactivity. The proteins contained another type of radioactivity. Then they allowed the virus to infect the bacteria.

Next, they put the mixture into the Waring Blendor and turned it on. The swirling solution knocked what remained of the viral particles off the bacteria. When they examined the bacteria, they only found radioactive DNA inside. The viral protein had remained on the outside of the bacteria and fell off once the blendor started. This told them that viral DNA got injected into the bacteria where it copied itself and gave rise to new viral particles. Thus, they confirmed DNA as the genetic material. A relatively simple experiment showed the central role of DNA in heredity. Hershey would share a Nobel Prize in 1969 for this discovery. Fred Waring, a popular musician, conductor, and radio-television personality, who invented the Waring Blendor, would not.

Further credence for the essential role of DNA came in 1953. James Watson and Francis Crick divined for the first time the spiral staircase structure of DNA and also garnered a Nobel Prize. But all these achievements failed to erase shadows obscuring how DNA directed the assembly of amino acids into proteins. Researchers termed the linking together chemically of amino acids into proteins "protein synthesis."

Scientists already knew that DNA resides majestically in a gated community in the cell called the nucleus. As the crux of the cell, DNA cannot risk the slightest damage to itself. So it must stay put. Yet, in the outer hinterlands (cytoplasm) of the cell, seemingly divorced from the nucleus, the making of protein rolls merrily along. So at the time of the Baltimore symposium, the largest missing pieces to the puzzle of life revolved around two issues: how could DNA in one location remotely direct the production of protein located in another? How could the four-letter structure of DNA lead to the 20-amino-acid structure of proteins?

Scientists would term this latter problem the issue of a "genetic code." DNA somehow held information in an encoded manner that got turned into the precise order of amino acids that distinguished one protein from another. Each protein was unique and contained a different arrangement of amino acids. How information in the spiral staircase structure of DNA gave rise to thousands of unique proteins in a cell constituted perhaps the greatest question in biology now facing scientists in the 20th century. Two years after leaving graduate school, Marshall would focus on that very question. To help answer it, he would have to learn much more about DNA and how amino acids were assembled into proteins.

At the time, scientists knew that RNA—a substance chemically similar to DNA—played a role in protein synthesis. Granules rich in ribosomal RNA and found in the cytoplasm of cells actively made protein. Whether other forms of RNA also participated in protein assemblage was anyone's guess.

Like others, Marshall struggled to understand how cells made proteins. His notebook entries referred to the ideas of George Gamow and others that DNA might physically serve as a pattern on which amino acids would fit and then be chemically zippered together. If this were the case, production of protein would have to occur *inside* the nucleus. Some scientists at the Baltimore symposium did, in fact conclude that "protein synthesis can occur in *both the nucleus* [italics added] and the cytoplasm … [the part of the cell outside the nucleus]."[3]

Only later would it become clear in that study that RNA granules from the cytoplasm clung to the nuclei and contaminated them. What appeared to be protein synthesis inside the nucleus was actually occurring on the attached RNA granules outside the nucleus. However, the suggestion that nuclei could also make protein gave Marshall a false illusion that proteins might physically be made directly on DNA. Marshall would pursue this mirage. He would try repeatedly to show that protein production could physically occur on top of DNA. He would initially overlook the possibility that DNA only serves as the source of information for how each protein is to be assembled.

Symposium participants in Baltimore wrangled over the details of protein production. Two ideas prevailed: one, that a class of proteins assembled a new protein by adding one amino acid at a time. The other idea envisioned some sort of pattern that the amino acids would attach to all at once.[4] The pattern might reside in the very structure of DNA or in a copy of DNA termed a messenger RNA. The messenger RNA would leave the nucleus. It would deliver directions to the cytoplasm where proteins got assembled.

But how to more easily study the ways cells make proteins? About 150 years earlier, scientists feared trying in their laboratories to duplicate organic molecules made in living organisms. They believed it could not be done. They reasoned that such molecules contained an "animating force" and could not be made by man. Eventually, scientists conquered their fear and showed the chemistry of life could be replicated in a laboratory.

Now more than a century later a similar challenge loomed. Could cells be ruptured and their pieces reassembled and made to work in test tubes? Or would some animating force be lost in the process? If rupture worked, the test tubes would be free of intact cells. The cell extracts would be referred to as "cell-free." Symposium participants now agreed that studies of protein production "demonstrated conclusively the value of cell-free preparations in elucidating the nature of the process of amino acid … [assembly into proteins]."[5]

Marshall took all this advice to heart. In Michigan, he had used intact cells from the abdomens of mice. Starting in 1959, he would switch instead to cells of bacteria. He saw, as did many others, that cell extracts offered some advantages. Cell extracts allowed a focus on one cell process at a time.

In addition, he could more clearly see what happens when he made one change or another.

The downside was not knowing how proteins actually got made inside a cell. To duplicate the process in a test tube, researchers had to guess: how much energy did the cell need to make protein? Did protein synthesis require sodium chloride, which is common table salt, or similar compounds? How long did it take for a cell to make a protein? What would be the best way to prepare the RNA granules (ribosomes) on which proteins appeared to be made? Seeking to optimize his system, Marshall would later "wash" the ribosomes and discover in the wash another form of RNA. This RNA would be the actual messenger that some had proposed. Others, however, would take credit away from Marshall for the same discovery.

In experiments that foreshadowed those of Marshall, researchers tried to see just what the role of DNA is. They reasoned that DNA is somehow directly involved in protein production. If so, then "knocking out" DNA should bring protein synthesis to a screeching halt. One way to "knock out" DNA is to add a protein called DNase, for short, to the cell extracts. DNase could reduce the spiral staircase structure of DNA to mere fragments. Loss of intact DNA structure would mean loss of function. When scientists eliminated DNA this way, protein synthesis still continued merrily along. However, even a partial loss of RNA was devastating. As far as the relationships between DNA, RNA, and protein, one presenter obliquely concluded, "The outlook is depressingly bright for quick resolution of many interesting problems."[6]

Virus too came into play. A virus that infected tobacco plants confirmed that RNA could also lead to synthesis of new virus.[7] "It will be a long time," said the study's author, "before anyone will attempt to decipher in chemical terms the code transmitting the 'information' carried by these relatively simple, and yet so formidable, [template] molecules."[7] In a few short years, Marshall would prove that prediction wrong.

Some thought a form of RNA might serve as a message for the making of protein. If so, they might tease out the arrangement of letters in RNA that specified a particular protein. Silk, with its unusually high amount of one particular amino acid, seemed a good candidate. Researchers could compare the RNA from cells making silk to the RNA from cells that did not. They expected to see in the messenger RNA for silk an abundance of one group of letters that specified the high amount of that one particular amino acid. That would then be the code word. But they saw no differences. The composition of silk messenger RNA appeared no different than that of the non-silk messenger RNA.[8] "This is not what we would expect at first sight if the triplet [a code consisting of three letters] idea was correct."[8]

In 1956, the authors could not yet know that they had simply looked at the total RNA from ribosomes. The letter composition of RNA from ribosomes does not vary much from cell to cell. Only a small fraction of RNA mixed in with the RNA from ribosomes is the actual messenger. Had they looked at just the messenger RNA from cells making silk, they would have likely seen the difference.

James Watson and Francis Crick also attended this conference. Crick thought that the postulated messenger RNA might be built two letters at a time rather than one.[9] Crick's position came under attack from Erwin Chargaff, embittered for having been passed over for his contributions to Watson and Crick's structural model for DNA. Chargaff had discovered that in DNA the ratios of A to T and G to C letters always equaled one. This finding had proved crucial for Watson and Crick's discovery of the structure of DNA. Chargaff chastised Crick, pointing out the difficulties with the two letter model. In contrast, Marshall held no preconceived view of either the construction of DNA and RNA or the number of letters in the genetic code needed to specify each amino acid. Rather, Marshall accepted whatever his data showed.

Marshall also read the paper by Severo Ochoa and Leon Heppel. Their study explored the use of a newly discovered protein assembling long chains of RNA.[10] Two years later, Ochoa would win a Nobel Prize for discovering this protein. The protein and the chains of letters it hooked together would figure heavily in Marshall's own discovery of the genetic code. As Marshall later stumbled toward his discovery, Ochoa would become one of his fiercest competitors. Heppel at NIH would become Marshall's equally fierce compatriot.

Marshall's future discovery of messenger RNA was presaged by another report. It found inside bacteria an RNA whose letter arrangement closely matched that of the DNA of the infecting virus. The commonality between DNA and this RNA became an early clue that the two might somehow be related.[11]

Marshall arrived at NIH in 1957 when the papers from this symposium came out in book form. That Marshall loved science and retained a boyish enthusiasm throughout his life for both research and the laboratory there is no doubt. But NIH could be an intimidating place for a young postdoctoral investigator. Marshall had received a solid, if somewhat stolid, education, first at the University of Florida and then at the University of Michigan. Those experiences still barely prepared him for the intellectual vigor and intensity of the people with top-notch educations that he now encountered at NIH. His mentor, Stetten, for example, had gone first to Harvard and then to medical school at Columbia. Gordon Tomkins, whose laboratory Marshall would shortly join, went to medical school at Harvard and then added a PhD degree from the University of California, Berkeley. Bill Jakoby, with whom Marshall studied proteins, used the very high level of training he received at Yale.

Daily events highlighted the differences between Marshall's training and those who now surrounded him. Marshall recalled a seminar at NIH by Fritz Lipmann, a biochemist who would eventually win the Nobel Prize. Marshall remembered:

Lipmann presented this discovery in … a … seminar, and … I … was appalled because that particular seminar group was a very tough group. They asked for the controls. "Did you do this control? Did you do that control?" The answer was "no" in all cases because this was a very early stage in the work. The evidence that he had was enough to convince me, but it sure wasn't enough to satisfy others. I never saw anything like it. He was virtually crucified. Of course, he was correct in everything that he said. That was a remarkable seminar.[12]

In his first two years at NIH, Marshall had failed to impress either Stetten or Jakoby. So Marshall, a very private person who did not reveal much about himself, likely felt he had something to prove. His personal notebooks are replete with jottings urging himself to work harder, work smarter, presumably just to keep up with others. These entries give the impression of his being haunted by memories of his father's struggles to make a living.

Marshall Meets a Mentor

By 1960, Marshall stood poised to help resolve both genetic code and protein synthesis questions. A remarkable man, Gordon Tomkins, would be Marshall's savior. Just as there are few men skilled at picking good horseflesh from a selection of young foals, Tomkins had the rare skill of discerning those few people early on who might later make a good run at a science career. Marshall became the first of Tomkins's such successes.

Marshall had met Tomkins at NIH early on. The two men attended a lunchtime seminar, a "journal club," in which participants debated the merits of recently published papers. Marshall regarded Tomkins as brilliant, a colleague whose unusual and original associations frequently made others laugh. Tomkins impressed people not only as a scientist but also as a musician so skilled that he played with one of the top bands of the era.[12]

Interestingly, Stetten felt confident that he, like Tomkins, knew how to review budding scientific talent. Recalled Bill Dryer, "DeWitt Stetten [then associate director of research at the National Institute of Arthritis and Metabolic Diseases, NIH] had been able to help identify extraordinary talent at the various labs. One of the things that he wrote and told me was that, when you are trying to recruit—as we are now in the Biology Division [at the California Institute of Technology]—when there's someone really extraordinary, it's just obvious. You're at a seminar and you know it. And that's what they had done at NIH."[13] Unlike Tomkins, though, Stetten completely misjudged Marshall's scientific talent. In this case, it was not so obvious to all.

Toward the end of 1959, Tomkins, recently appointed the head of an NIH lab, offered Marshall a position as an independent investigator. Tomkins had done the extraordinary. He had somehow divined in Marshall the exceptional man at a time when little stood out about Marshall as exceptional. In contrast, Stetten and Jakoby saw so little merit in Marshall that they made no effort to retain him. Perhaps in their meetings, Tomkins recognized that Marshall would go to almost unimaginable lengths to succeed. Unfortunately, there is no way to know how Tomkins made his decision. Tomkins died prematurely at age 49 following brain surgery.

Marshall said, "I wanted to do something completely different from what I had done before. I felt competent and ready to try to discover."[12] Marshall's desire for a challenge departed from some of his earlier decisions. As a graduate student at the University of Florida, Marshall worked in a groundbreaking laboratory that used radioisotopes to trace the pathways of life. But when it came to doing a master's thesis, he instead simply counted the caddis flies of Alachua County. Later, he chose to enter the University of Michigan despite acceptance at the stronger biochemistry department at the University of Wisconsin. Perhaps Marshall's decision now to strike out on his own represented the growing maturity of a 32-year-old man. Marshall may have also been further stimulated by the leading researchers and the high quality research being turned out then by the scientific staff of NIH.

Marshall's two main areas of interest lay in the direction of either the chemical basis of heredity or neurobiology—the study of the nervous system. He chose heredity, fearing it might be premature to enter neurobiology given how relatively little was known about the field. Besides, at the time, the discoveries being made about DNA, RNA, and the production of protein just seemed more exciting to him. Despite a total lack of experience with the chemical basis of heredity, Marshall took a deep breath and plunged in. The move entailed great risk to Marshall. The start of a scientific career requires rapid progress, creativity, and above all, publications. All would be hard to come by given his lack of knowledge about this whole area of research.

Marshall recalled, "One night, shortly after I became an independent investigator, I walked in the corridor adjacent to my lab and saw Bruce Ames, who was then one of the best scientists at the NIH. He was working at night in his lab, so on a whim I decided to ask his advice. I told him what my plans were as an independent investigator to determine whether m[essenger] is required for ... [use in cell extracts for] ... synthesis of a protein. When I told him this, he looked at me. He said, 'It's suicidal to do it.' So we both agreed that it would be extremely difficult and dangerous to work on this problem."[12]

Now 82 years old, Ames can't recall having that conversation. "I don't remember anything about that. It sounds sort of unlike me, but it came out in *Chemical Engineering News* ... that ... I told Marshall, 'It's way too complicated. Don't touch it,' and he ignored my advice and did this wonderful thing. Now, I'm usually very enthusiastic to people."[14]

So why did Marshall choose such a perilous path? He confessed being quite worried about it. He admitted he "wanted to play with the 'big boys,' with the best people in the field."[12] Perhaps the answer is more complex than that. Marshall had published papers during his two years with Jakoby. But both Jakoby and Stetten remained unimpressed and showed no interest in him.

Marshall either needed to forge a way to make a secure living or face having to return in embarrassment to Florida and life on the farm. He certainly wanted no part of that. Academic positions might have beckoned, but Marshall evinced no interest in them either. Even his new appointment with Tomkins came with strings attached. The position had not yet absolutely materialized, so Marshall had to remain a postdoctoral fellow. It was not a step up but rather one made laterally. Essentially, he had a year to prove himself.

Marshall still recalled the embarrassment of his father once asking Stetten whether Marshall could earn a decent living as a scientist.[12] Growing up, Marshall likely had inherited some of the angst of his father. Marshall claimed to be unconcerned about having a job. In reality, accepting the new position with Tomkins preserved Marshall's interest in being independent. But keeping it required making a big impact. So Marshall now concentrated on how DNA and, possibly, RNA, made protein production a reality.

Marshall began to teach himself all that he needed to know about DNA, RNA, and protein. He learned to speed read, improving to about 3,000 words per minute. But he found it of little use for the scientific literature, where he needed to review details carefully. Even so, Marshall managed to read at about 700 to 800 words a minute. But he also started going to professional meetings and learning more about biochemistry. The advances spurred on by the Watson-Crick discovery of DNA structure made research in the field seem electrically charged to a newcomer like Marshall.

Marshall had never taken a single course on the subject of DNA, RNA, and making of protein while a graduate student. To make up for that, he now enrolled in evening courses at NIH. Perhaps more importantly, Marshall realized that as his formal education had ended, he now needed to learn on his own. Self-instruction included reading the scientific literature, attending professional meetings, interacting with other professional scientists, and more reading of science. Marshall's lifelong habit of constantly reading science papers enabled him to pick up a small detail here or there that he might eventually find useful. Yet the self-teaching process was an imperfect one. Marshall would soon make a fundamental mistake, but one that would lead him to a Nobel Prize.

Penicillinase Opens a Door?

One summer, right at the beginning of Marshall's move to the Tomkins laboratory, both men attended a course on the genetics of bacteria at the Cold Spring Harbor Laboratory in Long Island, New York. There, they worked every day from 8:30 in the morning until midnight. Marshall learned how to make bacterial mutants, isolate DNA, and make extracts from cells. Marshall also found a way to test for a particular protein called penicillinase. His interest in penicillinase came from the fact that cells made it only at certain times. Production of this protein in bacteria had to be induced; otherwise, it remained absent from the cell.[12]

This training gave mixed results. It whet Marshall's appetite to learn more about this field. But later, it created a distraction when Marshall spent more time on getting intact cells to make penicillinase than on using cell extracts to make proteins. Penicillinase had to be made from scratch, when bacteria were properly induced; Marshall thought the hypothetical messenger RNA for the protein would suddenly appear when otherwise it would be absent. Marshall planned to isolate this presumed messenger RNA and determine the exact order of the letters in it. Then he would isolate penicillinase and determine the exact order of the amino acids making up this protein. Both the messenger RNA and protein were linear structures. He would line one up against the other. This would show him how many letters and which ones determined each amino acid in penicillinase. If successful, this experiment would unlock the code. It would show how a combination of four letters in messenger RNA could code for protein containing up to 20 different amino acids.[15]

Marshall knew that unlike most other proteins, penicillinase lacked a certain amino acid. Therefore, he would grow bacteria in the absence of that amino acid. Without that amino acid, the bacteria would be unable to make most proteins, which need it. But because penicillinase lacked that amino acid, its production would not stop. Marshall would then simply isolate both the messenger RNA and penicillinase protein and determine the order of the chemical building blocks of each.[12]

Marshall's idea was ahead of its time. Methods to determine the order of letters in RNA, the presumed messenger, did not yet exist. A method to determine the exact arrangement of amino acids in a protein had only recently been reported.[16]

Once in Tomkins's laboratory, Marshall found himself relegated to a side room where many of the large scientific instruments kept running. Although he had a laboratory bench that ran half the length of the space, the noise of one particular instrument in the room proved very distracting. Eventually, Marshall persuaded Tomkins to move the instrument to another location and to convert the room to a full research laboratory.[12] Despite these initial difficulties, Marshall said, "Working in Gordon's laboratory was a marvelous opportunity for me. I have never found anybody else that I could talk to in my entire life who really understood me."[12]

In late summer of 1959, Marshall began to extract from bacterial cells the components he needed in order to make proteins in a test tube. Marshall continuously scoured the scientific literature. Had he found a suitable paper in the scientific literature, he would have used the details as a starting point. Many people point to a paper in August 1960, as the key one.[17] The authors' names appear in Marshall's notes but not until the summer of 1960 when their paper first appeared.[18]

But Marshall started to prepare cell extracts a year before that publication appeared. This suggests he used details from another study to jumpstart his own work. A name that surfaces in Marshall's notes is that of Arthur Weissbach, another young scientist whom Marshall knew at NIH in the summer of 1959. Around the time that Marshall began to make cells extracts for studying the production of proteins, Weissbach did the same. He must have been ahead of Marshall because he published details of his work in

July 1960.[19] Marshall did not publish until nine months later. Marshall and Arthur Weissbach working in parallel at NIH likely discussed how best to make cell extracts capable of making new proteins in a test tube.

But Weissbach's methods contained a trap that Marshall adroitly avoided. Both men tracked the production of new protein by measuring how much of an added radioactive amino acid ended up in the protein. They first isolated the protein in their test tubes and then counted the amount of radioactivity in it. The more radioactivity they found in protein, the more new synthesis they assumed must have occurred.

This seemed quite straightforward. The method, however, was not foolproof. Mixed in with the radioactive protein might be, for example, droplets of the radioactive amino acid. If this occurred, they could easily overestimate the amount of new protein made. Marshall found that Weissbach's method gave lots of radioactivity in the protein fraction but did not give new protein. The tipoff, Marshall realized, came when he added antibiotics to his test tubes. The antibiotics should have blocked protein from being made but did not. Even in the presence of antibiotics, radioactivity continued to accumulate in the "protein" fraction. Clearly, in the presence of antibiotics, the enhanced radioactivity did not mark "true" production of new protein.

The discovery of soluble or sRNA highlighted the bright side of theory. But theory also held a dark side. Theory could illuminate research passageways that led nowhere. Marshall, occasionally blinded by the bright light of a theory stumbled about as he searched for the code.

In August 1960, for example, Marshall had remained captivated by Gamow's theory that DNA could serve as a direct template for protein synthesis. In fact, Marshall believed—later to be shown to be wrong—that nature commanded cells to make proteins two different ways. If cells used DNA as a physical pattern, Marshall could halt protein production by adding DNAse, a protein that destroyed DNA. This showed the need to keep DNA functional in the cell extracts. Similarly, he could treat extracts with a protein that destroyed RNA and also bring protein production to a stop. This pointed to the need to also have functional RNA.[20] It wasn't until November 1960 that Marshall realized that functional DNA might be needed to build the RNA messenger.[21] At the same time, Marshall noticed that he finally had a true increase in protein in his cell extracts. This production of protein continued unless he added an antibiotic to the cell extracts, and it continued in intact cells as well unless he added an antibiotic. For Marshall, the similar responses of intact cells and cell extracts to antibiotics marked a true measure of the making of proteins.[22]

Marshall and Tomkins involved themselves in quite disparate projects. Despite their differences, Tomkins knew the background and full details of Marshall's experiments. Lunchtime would find the two men discussing Marshall's latest progress and the exciting results just published by others. Marshall recalled Tomkins coming in to talk, slouching up against the refrigerator with a sandwich in one hand. A shorthand form of speaking transpired in which each man could sense where the other might be headed. Before one could finish, the other would cut in and anticipate the answer. The resulting conversation would be rapid-fire. But Tomkins would literally pin Marshall down if he said something illogical or wrong. Out of these daily exchanges, ideas flowed and got batted around.[12]

In these discussions, Marshall's thoughts ranged far and wide. Yet his inexperience showed a lack of discipline and focus needed to solve the genetic code problem. In September 1959, for example, Marshall's notebook entries swung breathlessly from whether RNA and DNA could be used to alter cells to how the three-dimensional structure of proteins formed; what happens to mice infected by a virus; whether protein synthesis affected learning in monkeys; the biological conditions needed to make penicillinase; whether steroids could pass through the placenta of pregnant women; and whether fingerprints could be transferred genetically.[23–30] It was too much to think about.

Marshall became especially interested in the reported discovery of sRNA. It appeared to transport amino acids to ribosomes, the site for protein production. There, sRNA might also align the amino acids on a template in the same order as they appeared in the finished protein. Thus, this sRNA appeared to be the adaptor molecule previously postulated.[31]

Marshall entered the field of the chemical basis of heredity just as other key discoveries began to emerge. François Jacob and Jacques Monod reported on what controls how genes express information that results in the making of new protein.[32] The production of protein seemed to take place on RNA particles that made up ribosomes. Studies had confirmed that assumption.[33] All these discoveries would figure in Marshall's work as he tried to duplicate in his test tubes how living cells made proteins.

Using cell extracts gave Marshall more control of the protein-making process than would be possible with intact cells. Marshall also knew of published suggestions that yet a third type of RNA might also be involved in protein production. This unknown RNA could bridge the gap between DNA inside the nucleus and the making of proteins outside. The RNA might serve as a messenger to bring information encoded in DNA to ribosomes. There, the information would be used to make new protein.

Marshall recalled, "I thought that ... [messenger RNA] ... might be contained in ribosomes because amino acids were known to be ... [assembled] ... into protein on ... [ribosomes] .... I estimated that it would take two years to set up ... [cell extracts] ... to determine whether RNA or DNA stimulated protein synthesis. It did ... [take that long]."[34]

Despite knowing little about bacteria and even less about protein synthesis, Marshall plunged ahead. This was no easy matter. A host of experimental details had to be worked out, and hard planning decisions made. Marshall would, for example, need to distinguish the true production of protein from false production. How best to tell what was occurring? Studies with the protein penicillinase could help. Induction would cause bacteria to make penicillinase and its messenger RNA where none would otherwise be present. Marshall could use a radioactive amino acid to track production of the protein.

What exactly did Marshall need to add to the cell extracts to optimize protein production? On which protein should he first focus his attention? Protein production requires energy: what energy source would work best? Would sRNA be needed and, if so, how much? Would he also have to add the chemical building blocks needed to make more RNA?[35] How could ribosomes best be isolated, purified, and stored?[36,37] Would the "cell sap" remaining after the collection of ribosomes be useful?[38]

Marshall complicated his approach by trying to use two different types of bacteria at one time: one to induce the production of penicillinase in intact bacteria and the other to make proteins using extracts of cells. Although the production of penicillinase by inducing it in bacterial cells gave him trouble, Marshall persisted in getting it to work.[39] Working on two different projects, not surprisingly, proved difficult. Each called for different methods and handling. Thus, Marshall's attention to one repeatedly diverted his attention to the other. As a result, progress on both slowed. Once protein production stopped in both systems, Marshall sped the work up by adding an acid to the test tubes. The acid caused protein to drop out of solution. Then Marshall collected the protein and determined its radioactivity.

Marshall likely borrowed Weissbach's use of filters to easily capture newly made protein in the cell extracts. Marshall then placed the filter in a small glass container and placed it in a radioactivity counter.[40] Marshall possibly borrowed other details as well, which was perfectly normal. Marshall added a chemical to stabilize the cell extract and keep it active as did Weissbach. Others did not. Marshall, like Weissbach, simply measured the amount of radioactivity in the proteins. Others laboriously measured both the radioactivity and the actual amount of protein. Weissbach meticulously toyed with conditions for his system: amount of ribosomes to be added, amount of "cell sap" containing the sRNA and other components, length of time to run a reaction, and other details. Marshall followed suit. Weissbach raised the amount of magnesium salt over what had been used before. Marshall raised it still further.

Doing these experiments in the space Tomkins gave him energized Marshall and reinforced his desire for independence. He reminisced, "At that time, in 1960, the work was getting very exciting. I don't think I took any vacations. I may have gone for a weekend to the beach, but I don't remember any vacation. That was my life. I just worked: that was all. I went out on dates and to parties, but this was what my life was."[12]

Shortly after, Marshall began to record what he mistakenly regarded as his cell extracts successfully making new protein. The material on his filters, which he assumed to be protein, contained the expected radioactivity. But was the radioactive amino acid actually attached in the protein or just hanging out on the filter? Tests with antibiotics soon confirmed what he dreaded to admit: no true production.

Marshall had decided before that the gold standard for producing new protein would be its sensitivity to added antibiotics. Now when he added antibiotics to his own test tubes, he continued to find radioactively labeled protein on his filters. True protein production would have stopped. His cell extracts were producing nothing more than disappointment.[41]

Marshall knew that his cell extracts still contained DNA. A key question for Marshall remained the role of this DNA in his test tubes. Did DNA act like a copy machine, making copies of itself in the form of messenger RNA? Marshall thought two possibilities existed for the role of DNA: one, DNA itself acted as the physical pattern on which new protein got made. If so, he could destroy DNA in his test tubes by adding another protein called DNase, which literally "chews" up DNA into unusable fragments. When Marshall added DNase, the making of protein might cease. Alternatively, the production of new protein did not involve DNA directly. In that case, after adding the protein DNase, new protein would still be made. That would then suggest that messenger RNA, not DNA, functioned directly to make new protein.[42]

The possibility that messenger RNA participated directly in making new protein intrigued Marshall. He might be able to discard the natural messenger in his cell extracts and substitute an unnatural messenger in its place. A simple unnatural messenger would consist of a long chain of just one chemically linked-together letter, such as UUUUUUUUUUU.[43] Each "U" was one of the four chemical building blocks making up RNA.

Thus, for the first time, Marshall toyed with the idea of replacing natural messenger RNA with an unnatural messenger RNA. The unnatural messenger RNA could possibly reveal how a combination of letters in RNA directs the order of amino acids in proteins. It could tell him what amino acids enter new protein when directed by the unnatural messenger. Less than three years had elapsed since Marshall first thought about "cracking" the code.[44]

The plethora of different forms of RNA in cells complicated Marshall's efforts to understand how proteins got made. There were the ribosomes that acted as the site for making protein. Added to that was the sRNA that transported amino acids to the ribosomes. Now there might be a messenger RNA too. Adding the protein DNase to his cell extracts, Marshall found, gave mixed results. Sometimes the production of protein stopped and sometimes it did not. It depended, in part, on who had given him the DNase. Later, he would find that the protein DNase might be contaminated with another protein that destroyed RNA. Despite the confusing results, these experiments encouraged Marshall to examine the activities of both natural and unnatural messenger RNA in his cell extracts.[45]

On November 4, 1960, Marshall again speculated on preparing an unnatural messenger RNA to see whether it perhaps would also attach to ribosomes, just as natural messenger RNA might do. Attachment to ribosomes might be necessary in order for the ribosomes to participate in producing new protein.[46]

There were other questions to also be considered. Would the RNA of ribosomes, sRNA, and messenger RNA all be needed for the production of proteins in his test tubes?[47] To answer that question, Marshall would have to separate out the actions of a hypothetical messenger RNA from the actions of the RNA of ribosomes and sRNA. Each RNA might be expected to play a different role in making new protein. Most critical of all, however, was whether Marshall could trust cells extracts to provide answers to what actually went on in intact cells.[48]

Matthaei Joins Marshall

In October 1960, a recent postdoctoral newcomer to NIH from Germany named Johannes Heinrich Matthaei joined Marshall's lab. Two years younger than Marshall, Matthaei was handsome, slender, and cultured. It would prove to be an interesting pairing: the German with precise handwriting, bearing, and manner with the American whose handwriting could be indecipherable, his bearing ruffled, and a gracious manner with southern charm. Matthaei had become interested in plant biology when only three or four years old. That interest grew under outstanding biology teachers both in high school (known as "the gymnasium" in Germany) and college. After college, Matthaei experimented with how plants made proteins. Following up on this work and graduate study lured him eventually to America.

Armed with a NATO Research Fellowship, Matthaei came to the United States determined to apply to plants the most current knowledge of how bacteria and animals cells made protein. But his search would initially prove futile. He first arrived as a NATO Fellow at Cornell University, in upstate New York. There he found his mentor no longer interested in the proposed project before it even began. Discouraged but persistent, Matthaei, in September 1960, headed off to New York City. He hoped to team up with Nobel Laureate Fritz Lipmann. But Lipmann had no room in his laboratory. Then on to the Wister Institute in Philadelphia to work with internationally known biochemist and biophysicist Britton Chance. But again out of luck. Chance was not interested.

Receiving a lead, and having recently learned how to drive, Matthaei traveled down to NIH in an old 1951 Cadillac. Matthaei thought that with all the research at NIH, some people must be using cell extracts to make protein. But on arriving, he was surprised to learn there was just one: Marshall.[34] "Obviously," said Matthaei, "Marshall Nirenberg was the person I was looking for."[49] Tomkins agreed to the arrangement, and Matthaei transferred to Bethesda shortly before November 1. Matthaei later learned that half of all NATO Research Fellows had to switch for one reason or another to a different guest laboratory once in the United States. So his experience was not unusual.

From January 1960 onward, Marshall had focused on making his cell extracts work better in a test tube. He varied his methods for bashing open the bacterial cells. He searched for the best way to gently but fully remove the cell contents. He pulled various chemicals off the shelf to help "clean up" the ribosomes. Newly made proteins appeared on the ribosomes. He threw into his system a variety of antibiotics and watched them block the synthesis of proteins. Day after day, experiment after experiment, Marshall probed and tested, experimented and noted. After each full day of lab work, Marshall relaxed by wading through piles of the latest scientific papers. The next day, he returned to the lab. "Hurry up experiments," he wrote. "Should take 1 week to know whether system will work. Work—work—work. ...Get the answer fast."[50]

Meanwhile, two of the RNA Tie Club members, Francis Crick and Sydney Brenner, devised a three-point hypothesis about the postulated RNA messenger. Because they were still of two minds about the ideas, they declined to publish the document.[51]

The three hypothetical points about the messenger included:

1. Most of the RNA of ribosomes is not messenger RNA
2. Messenger RNA has the same letter ratios (A:U and G:C) as DNA
3. Messenger RNA (under some circumstances at least) is unstable and is destroyed. If destroyed then the messenger RNA is quickly remade.

Despite nailing the as-yet unseen messenger, Crick and Brenner did not immediately hammer out a paper to support it. Virtually at the same time, Marshall, who was not privy to this correspondence, independently came up with the same idea that ribosomes held two different types of RNA.[52]

Recalled Marshall:

I thought that if m[essenger] RNA existed, then some [messenger] RNA would be present on ribosomes. I had also prepared DNA. ... Matthei and I were determining the effect of adding DNA or ribosomal RNA on ... radioactive amino acid] ... incorporation into protein in the cell ... [extracts] ... from E. coli. After supper, I came back to the lab to see the preliminary results. The addition of ... [messenger] RNA stimulated the incorporation of ... [radioactivity] ... into protein, whereas adding DNA had no effect. The radioactivity counts were very low, but the duplicates agreed well and all the controls were present. I shouted and jumped in the air for joy because this was the first evidence that m[essenger] RNA, rather than DNA, directs the synthesis of protein. All of our subsequent work on deciphering the genetic code was a logical extension of that experiment."[53]

Marshall and Matthaei then relentlessly pursued their idea until they became the first to draw messenger RNA out from the ribosomes.[54] As Nobel Laureate Fritz Lipmann put it, "Things are moving very fast suddenly and this fellow Nirenberg has given us a good push."[55]

Marshall's and Matthaei's first paper led to the first proof of messenger RNA. Submitted on March 22, 1961, they reported they had "washed" the ribosomes. When they did so, natural messenger RNA ended up in the wash fluid. The ribosomes no longer had the needed directions for making protein. No protein got made as a result. However, when they added the messenger RNA back to the ribosomes, protein production resumed.[56] Marshall and Matthaei realized that this messenger RNA might be the pattern on which sRNA arranged the order of amino acids into proteins. But how the pattern encoded information left the two authors in the dark.

It took about another two months for members of the RNA Tie Club to catch up to Marshall and Matthaei's discovery of messenger RNA. The previously imagined messenger RNA now had become a reality. It explained how information from DNA in the nucleus directed the ribosomes in the cytoplasm to make proteins. Two members of the RNA Tie Club confirmed Marshall and Matthaei's discovery. Watson, who with Crick had discovered the structure of DNA, was one.[57] Brenner was the other.[58]

The first round had been fired in the battles to come over the genetic code. A furious race with Marshall, still somewhat fresh out of graduate school, stood poised to begin. Both Watson and Brenner—one on the verge of the Nobel Prize and the other later to be anointed Nobel Laureate—would lead a scientific assault on priority for discovering messenger RNA and the size of each "word" in the genetic code.

Showing for the first time the existence of messenger RNA provided Marshall with a critical insight. Removing messenger RNA from ribosomes gave him an idea. If natural messenger RNA could be *removed* from ribosomes, why couldn't an unnatural messenger RNA be *added back* in its place? If that proved possible, he could measure which amino acid(s) the unnatural messenger directed into protein.[43] If either Watson or Brenner from their studies on messenger RNA had the same idea, they failed to follow up on it.

Marshall and Matthaei's experiments proved time-consuming and difficult. It took about two full days just to make the cell extracts. Sometimes the extracts worked and sometimes they didn't. Even extracts that worked before might not work again after storage in a deep freezer. Marshall and Matthaei initially made up the radioactive amino acids used in the experiments. They did not buy them. Once used up, the radioactive amino acids had to be prepared again. Coils of paper tape recorded numbers of radioactivity that then had to be used in calculations, tables, and graphs. Repeating experiments often gave disparate results.[59]

Frustrated, Marshall wrote to himself, "Find out what is going on quickly and then decide whether or not to continue it. Stop fooling around. Should be able to do a table ... [of data] ... a day. Grind out results for paper in workaholic fashion."[60]

But what about the role of DNA? Marshall now came up with a new experimental wrinkle: he would mask the DNA in the cell extracts, thereby rendering it useless. He would find materials to physically attach to DNA, making it unable to function. By doing so Marshall, once and for all, could rule out DNA in the making of protein. He considered two possible ways to obscure the DNA. One consisted of adding a long chain of sugars chemically hooked together. The sugars would be electrically inert, i.e., would not carry any positive or negative charge. The other added separately would consist of a chemically linked chain of A's, one of the building blocks of natural RNA, such as AAAAAAAAAAAAAA, that carried negative charges.[61]

In the early 1950s, when the structure of DNA remained unclear, some thought it might consist of three chains rather than two. Perhaps Marshall thought so too when he expected AAAAAAAAAAAAAA to cling to DNA. However, Watson and Crick had already proven a three-chain structure false for natural DNA. AAAAAAAAAAAAAA would also not form such a structure with DNA.[62] Thus, adding it to prevent DNA from acting was doomed from the start. But it would surprisingly give Marshall and Matthaei a clue on how the code worked.[63]

Marshall also chose the wrong radioactive amino acid for this experiment. However, he had no way to know yet that it would not respond to AAAAAAAAAAAAAA. All seemingly went well at first. The two thousand units of radioactivity on the filters showed that true production of new protein occurred. Adding the protein DNAase cut the amount of radioactivity into new protein down to 800 units. This indicated that loss of DNA led to loss of new protein. Adding both DNase and AAAAAAAAAAAAAA, a double threat to DNA, reduced levels of radioactivity in protein further. So good, so far. These numbers supported Marshall's hypothesis of DNA involvement.

Only one number disturbed him. It occurred when he added just AAAAAAAAAAAAAA to the cell extracts. Marshall expected it would cover DNA and prevent the production of protein. In that case, the amount of radioactivity in protein should go down. To his surprise, the amount of radioactivity went up instead. It did not go up by much, a mere 20 percent. Many researchers might have overlooked such a small change. They might have felt that simply repeating the exact same experiment over and over again would show a 20 percent fluctuation. One would never get exactly the same amount of radioactivity in protein each time. The use of cell extracts remained somewhat of an art.

However, Marshall's greatest strength as a scientist lay in experimenting rather than in theory. He did not merely assume fluctuation. He insisted on tirelessly repeating the experiment time-after-time to see just how much actual variation occurred. Marshall's intuition suggested these data indicated something unusual. Perhaps AAAAAAAAAAAAAA had directed the synthesis of 20 percent more protein. This idea conflicted directly with his original assumption that it could *interfere* with DNA directing the making of protein. The difference between what he expected and what he got when he added AAAAAAAAAAAAAA tied Marshall's thoughts in knots.

As would be true for the next several years, at least, serendipity—the art of making a discovery when searching for something else—shadowed Marshall. Even today, more than 50 years later, why Marshall and Matthaei got these results is unclear. AAAAAAAAAAAAAA should not have directed the amino acid they used into protein. Somehow it did. Most likely, either AAAAAAAAAAAAAA or the amino acid held a contaminant. One or the other impurity might then enable radioactivity to go into the protein.

The 20 percent result was still too small for Marshall and Matthaei to claim a discovery. They felt compelled to further explore this odd result. On January 13, 1961, Marshall and Matthaei tottered on the edge of scientific immortality. Unknowingly, they were about to witness for the first time how in their cell extracts a genetic code worked. Instead of attention on DNA, they now focused on this unnatural messenger RNA. Marshall thought of using all 18 radioactive amino acids together in cell extracts separately with AAAAAAAAAAAAAA, GGGGGGGGGGGGGG, CCCCCCCCCCCCCC, and UUUUUUUUUUUUUU. They would check if any one of these markedly increased new protein as indicated by uptake of radioactivity into protein. If so, they would methodically go back and check to find, one by one, which amino acid(s) were involved. The first step to deciphering the genetic code would soon be at hand.[64]

However, Marshall took no chances. Unable to predict what might happen, he remained conservative. Marshall searched for a simple natural messenger RNA to add to cell extracts. Meanwhile, Matthaei worked on using the unnatural messenger RNA. Marshall found that RNA from tobacco mosaic virus was 30 to 50 times more active than ribosomal RNA at stimulating amino acid incorporation into protein. He arranged to go to California for further studies on this natural RNA messenger. Marshall recalled, "I felt like Marco Polo exploring a new area."[34]

Back at NIH, Matthaei found the levels of radioactivity in protein jumped when he added UUUUUUUUUUUUUU to the cell extracts. However, he was using all 18 different radioactive amino acids at the same time. They now had to find whether all the amino acids or just one was being directed into the new protein being made. Running experiment after experiment, Matthaei systematically whittled the group of 18 amino acids down to find out which one(s) were ending up in protein.

Matthaei remembers:

I was total[ly] excited foreseeing the expected result, enjoing [sic] working through the nights. The unusual activity of ... [UUUUUUUUUUUUUU] ... I knew from the first ... experiment ... with the C^{14} amino acid mix on May 21. So I spent the days May 22-27 testing the amino acids in groups (to save ... [UUUUUUUUUUUUUU] ... of which I only had 1 milligram and had used much more than necessary in the first pilot ... experiment ... doing everything in duplicate). The final alternative for decision on May 27 at 3:00 a.m. was either tyrosine or phenylalanine."[65]

The new results seemed indisputable. They had added a radioactive amino acid called phenylalanine to cell extracts devoid of natural messenger RNA. The radioactive counts in new protein stood at only 44. Then they threw in the unnatural messenger UUUUUUUUUUUUUU. The radioactivity in protein jumped a thousand times higher. Marshall and Matthaei had discovered that UUUUUUUUUUUUUU acted as an unnatural "messenger RNA."[66]

The unnatural messenger RNA directed the synthesis of a protein containing just that one amino acid. That meant that some combination of "U's" formed a code word for the amino acid phenylalanine. Just how many U's made up the code word? Some researchers had predicted the number would be 3, but they had to admit "we cannot be certain that the coding ratio is not 6."[67] In fact, it could have even been 9! Regardless, Marshall now had a way to look for coding of other amino acids. Marshall and Matthaei had finally "cracked" the code.

Fifty years later, the events surrounding this experiment remain indelibly etched in Matthaei's mind:

The morning after the night of final discovery, I met Gordon Tompkins around 9[am], when he came in. It required just ... grateful laughing and ... few words reporting success, including the enormous stimulation for [the amino acid phenylalanine] above background. ... Of course I had spoken to him the day before, how I would now approach the final decision between ... [checking the final two possible amino acids]... tyrosine and phenylalanine. Probably this made Gordon curious to come in on a Saturday morning. ... Gordon kept it secret for months, although he went to most relevant conferences."[68]

While Matthaei made this finding, Marshall had gone to California. Marshall recalled that after spending a month there, he received a call from Matthaei. Matthaei excitedly told Marshall that UUUUUUUUUUUUUU directed just one of the possible 20 amino acids into protein. Marshall wasted no time in flying back to Bethesda.[34]

However, Marshall and Matthaei remained concerned that no one would believe that their strange protein contained only one amino acid. But how to show this? Proteins usually contain a combination of amino acids. Fortunately, in a neighboring lab there luckily appeared one person most likely to know. Michael Sela worked with unusual protein materials. He knew that Marshall and Matthaei's strange protein, if correctly identified, would dissolve only if special acids were used. When Marshall and Matthaei tested their product, it behaved exactly as expected[34]

When Marshall later went to Moscow to announce at an international meeting their success, Matthaei also showed that CCCCCCCCCCCCCC directed just one amino acid—a different one—into protein.[34]

But cracking the genetic code also produced cracks in the relationship between Marshall and Matthaei. Separated by a scant two years of age, Matthaei chafed under Marshall's leadership. At the same time, Matthaei says he felt conflicted about staying. After Marshall later presented their results in Moscow in the summer of 1961, Marshall would decide to compete against recent Nobel Laureate Severo Ochoa for priority on discovering the code. Marshall therefore would accept a bevy of new research associates into his lab.

Matthaei felt protective about their recent discovery to which he had richly contributed. He looked aghast at the crowded laboratory. He says, the unnatural messengers they had stored there became unusable when the inexperienced new workers used contaminated pipettes. "I lost control ... [of] ... our lab['s] policy, decided to work from 5:00 p.m. to 8:00 a.m., repe[a]ted all results of the others myself to be sure; but ... [Marshall] ... would not trust my results correcting errors of others any more.[69]

Despite the enormous significance of his work with Marshall, Matthaei says he did not consider extending his fellowship or seeking other support.[69] Recalls Matthaei, "I wanted to establish a new lab as soon as possible to get working on deciphering the coding sequences. ... In the moment of discovery of coding ... it appeared just perfect to us. Exactly what one had hoped for. We were lucky ... throughout the entire deciphering of the code ... The really reliable, final evidence would come only later when many ... proteins and their genes could be compared in various organisms."[70]

In April 1961, Matthaei left with his family for a roundtrip to California and then back to New York City. On the way, he gave a dozen invited lectures. In the process, Matthaei wore out his used Cadillac, and reluctantly gave it to a junkyard. In New York, the family boarded the ship, Berlin, and arrived 10 days later at Bremerhaven, Germany. First invited by Nobel Laureate Max Delbrück to join his new Institute of Genetics in Cologne, Matthaei eventually accepted a two-year position at the Max Planck Institute of Biology in Tubingen. He then planned to take up an Associate Professorship in Cleveland, Ohio, but later opted to remain in Germany.

Max Delbrück was an eventual Nobel Laureate who led the phage group and held membership in the RNA Tie Club. Matthaei told Delbrück of their success. Delbrück loudly voiced his doubts that Marshall and Matthaei, two outliers of the scientific enterprise, could have discovered the genetic code.[71] Matthaei addressed Delbrück's queries as honestly as possible only to be stung by Delbrück's retort, "You are not candid." Greatly disappointed, Matthaei realized that Delbrück's view of leading a collection of scientists differed fundamentally from his own of a congenial collaboration or complete independence. Undeterred, Matthaei stated, "[I had a] strong conviction, my discoveries … would … turn out to be useful for science and humanity."[71]

The use of unnatural messenger RNA UUUUUUUUUUUUU opened a path to the genetic code. For Marshall, the discovery marked not an end but a difficult beginning. Like David facing Goliath, Marshall would eventually be forced against great odds to defend his discovery with Matthaei. But first he had to announce it to the world.

8   The Cold War

In August of 1961, Marshall along with Matthaei perched on the cusp of a biological revolution. Marshall was scheduled to give a talk at the International Congress of Biochemistry in Moscow. Just before leaving for Russia, he married Perola Zaltzman, a biochemist from Rio de Janeiro who also worked at NIH. The two had met when they both lived on the NIH campus in the same building and had adjoining apartments.[1] The couple planned to meet for a leisurely, two-week honeymoon after the meeting.

The meeting in Moscow occurred at the height of the Cold War with Russia, which extended from 1947 to 1991. In August 1961, the West rebuffed the Soviet Union's demand to leave West Berlin. In response, East Berlin erected the infamous Berlin Wall to stem the flow of East Germans trying to escape Communism by crossing over to the West sector.

Fifteen months earlier, the United States had been embarrassed when a high altitude spy plane had been shot down while monitoring Soviet nuclear arms activity. As a result, a scheduled meeting between President Eisenhower and Soviet leader Nikita Khrushchev was canceled after President Eisenhower explained that the plane was an off-course weather plane. In fact, Khrushchev had withheld news that the pilot had survived along with enough debris to identify the plane's spyware.

Four months before the Congress, a Soviet cosmonaut, Yuri Gagarin, had orbited the Earth in Vostok 1 and returned safely. The streets of Moscow remained littered with placards bearing his portrait. It would be another eight years before the United States caught up to the Soviet Union in the space race.[2]

Fortunately, the Biochemistry Congress itself proved more peaceful, as scientists attended from 58 different countries. A. I. Oparin, president of the Biochemical Society of the U.S.S.R., in the opening session, presciently commented, almost as if here were talking directly to Marshall, "Youth is our future. The fate of the science to which we have dedicated our lives is in their hands. ... I would like to hope that this Congress will remain in the hearts of these young people as one of the most important events in their scientific lives."[3]

Marshall Makes His Mark

Marshall may not have realized at that moment that he was about to assume a mantle of scientific leadership. His scheduled presentation bore little resemblance to the benign abstract previously submitted in advance of the meeting. Some 6,000 people attended. The organizers had invited more than half of the 3,500 foreign scientists to present their findings. Marshall was just one of many. He had missed the symposium in Baltimore five years earlier. Now he was about to step onto a world stage at the Congress in Moscow.

Bernard Agranoff, who met Marshall in Moscow, remembered nervous jokes among the Western European and American attendees about being followed or rooms that might have been bugged. Despite the Cold War, no major political flaps occurred. Stolid, humorless representatives of Intourist, the official (and only) Soviet travel agency, handled travel or accommodation issues. Passports were collected and not returned until the meeting ended.[2]

Marshall knew some of the other attendees at the Congress. Minor J. Coon from the Department of Biological Chemistry at Michigan came as did Gordon Tomkins and many others from NIH. But neither Coon nor Tomkins had any interest in the technicalities of Marshall's presentation. Marshall later expressed disappointment that only 35 people initially attended his announcement of an experiment with unnatural messenger. But it should not have come as a surprise. Marshall and Matthaei had submitted their abstract well in advance of the Congress. The abstract made no mention of an unnatural messenger directing the production of protein or even a single thing about the genetic code.

Rather, their abstract spoke of an odd way their cell extracts made protein. Some new protein appeared even when they left out ribosomes. The ribosomes were the sites in the cell extracts on which newly made protein first appeared. Current knowledge even then held that the production of proteins required ribosomes. But the authors also acknowledged that part of their cell extracts did depend on ribosomes and did "have many characteristics of protein synthesis."[4] Other labs also focused on the use of cell extracts to make proteins in test tubes. So Marshall and Matthaei's abstract revealed no striking new discovery and, in fact, at least one discrepancy with current understanding.

However, in the interim between abstract submission and the start of the Congress, Marshall and Matthaei had made a startling discovery that became the real point of their presentation. The two authors had substituted for naturally occurring messenger an unnatural messenger, UUUUUUUUUUUUU. The unnatural messenger RNA had directed the making of a protein containing just one amino acid. The experiment indicated a long-awaited breakthrough in deciphering the genetic code. It indicated how the combination of letters in DNA might encode information for the order of amino acids in proteins. The experiment signaled a first step in assembling a dictionary of genetic code words. It revealed that some combinations of the letter U directed the insertion of the amino acid phenylalanine into protein.

The Congress took place in Lomonosov Moscow State University, about 200 years old at the time. The University's gargantuan campus hosted a bewildering mélange of 1,000 buildings and structures. The marginally functional meeting venue and accommodations basically consisted of Moscow University classrooms and student dormitories. Attendees reached the classrooms through a labyrinth of hallways that wended their way through the massive building in which the Congress was held.

Marshall presented in a classroom made even darker by the absence of windows. Instead, rows of fluorescent lights cast a garish glow. Long wooden desks and benches crowded the room. The Soviet slide projectors used large lantern slides and lacked zoom lenses, but most speakers had only brought 35 mm slides. "Consequently," recalled Agranoff, "the speakers had to refer to postage stamp–sized images projected on a bed-sheet screen to describe their research presentations."[2]

Attendance at the smaller sessions dwindled. "Like most of us," Agranoff recalled, "Marshall was disappointed that his striking discovery would go unnoticed. I saw him ... [later] ... on the street near the meeting hall, and he dispiritedly suggested taking a break ... [from the meeting] ... and visiting the mausoleum in Red Square, where the refrigerated remains of both Lenin and Stalin were on display."[2]

Matthew Meselson, then a young professor at Harvard University, attended Marshall's presentation. Some 50 years later he can't recall exactly why. "Something about the title intrigued me, but ... the title was innocuous. ... But I heard his talk, and I was so moved by it. After he had finished, I ran up, and I actually hugged him. I don't think I kissed him, but I really embraced him strongly."[5]

Meselson recalls that after hearing Marshall's talk, he "went running around—literally running around the halls trying to find Francis [Crick]. … Francis was clearly the dominant figure of the meeting, in my opinion. And I knew that he would have the clout to have the organizers have Marshall talk to a plenary session. … I told … [Crick] … that Marshall had some … [unnatural messenger] … RNA, and they made specific amino acids be incorporated in the ribosome system. And, of course, Crick understood that instantaneously."[5] As a result of Crick's intervention, Marshall addressed the Congress again, this time to a sizable group worthy of hearing Marshall's announcement.

Marshall felt grateful for Meselson's reaction. Marshall later recounted that it had meant a lot to him, more than all kinds of awards, because it seemed so genuine and spontaneous. Remembering his own reaction, Marshall later made it a point to try to congratulate people in his own laboratory in a similarly spontaneous and sincere way.[6]

Nobel Laureate Severo Ochoa attended this second presentation. Ochoa went running out of the room where Marshall was talking, telegraphed his group, and told them to get on it immediately.[7]

Hugs aside, the real coin of the science realm is unquestionably priority: who is the first to make a discovery. On the slim difference between a submission date affixed to one scientific paper or another, an entire career can rest. Announcing the results at the Congress in Moscow placed Marshall in a delicate dilemma. Marshall had established priority to the discovery. But that now left him exposed to very serious competition. Scientists believed the genetic code—the language of biological life—consisted of 64 different letter combinations. Marshall's presentation had revealed only *one* of the possible letter combinations. Like a baby's first word, the discovery signaled the start to understanding the language of biology. Scientists acting as linguists would now race to uncover the other 63 letter combinations that made up this newly discovered language.

Scientists like Nobel Laureate Severo Ochoa could draw on vastly more experience than Marshall had. Others might have more research funds and laboratory staff. They would use Marshall and Matthaei's discovery as a springboard for the mental gymnastics needed to find more letter combinations. Marshall would easily be left behind before he had barely left the starting gate.

If another scientist managed to decipher the rest of the code, Marshall and Matthaei would be relegated at best to an historical footnote. No book would likely ever likely be written about them. Supplanting them, the eventual winner would become a prime candidate to win the holy grail of

science, namely the Nobel Prize. Marshall's inexperience and youth, location at a government laboratory rather than an academic one, and limited resources immediately branded him the dark horse in the race to succeed. Marshall had to publish results quickly to stake his claim. But the more he published, the more details of the work he would gave away to his competitors. Then they could potentially surpass him.

Given the excitement Marshall's second presentation generated, he should have returned directly to his lab. "I thought," said Marshall, "that was the worst time in the world to take a vacation, but I felt that you only get married once, and it was worth it."[6] Marshall really didn't really have enough money for marriage. As a postdoctoral fellow, he made $3,000 a year. He had not fared much better after joining Tomkins's lab because they had no position immediately available. Therefore, Marshall had to accept yet another postdoctoral appointment. Fortunately, his wife Perola had saved some money, which made the honeymoon possible.[6]

Linda Greenhouse, Marshall's first lab technician, remembers that Marshall "always was a very handsome guy, charming, very handsome, and ... the girls at NIH, the unmarried, they were after him, that's for sure. And all of a sudden he comes in one day and says, 'I got married.' Nobody knew who she was, and it was like where did this come from? It was really funny but that's Marshall."[8]

Marshall and Matthaei sought publication in one of the most prestigious science journals in the world, the *Proceedings of the National Academy of Sciences of the United States*. The paper had to be communicated to the journal by a member of the Academy. Yet, Marshall had trouble getting the paper published. He submitted it to several people including the great atomic physicist, Leó Szilárd. Szilárd said he did not understand the paper and declined to submit it. NIH again came to the rescue. Joseph E. Smadel, chief of the Laboratory of Virology and Rickettsiology at the Division of Biologics Standards at NIH communicated the groundbreaking paper. Neither Marshall nor Matthaei at the time had yet been elected to membership in the National Academy of Sciences.

Marshall had not a moment to lose. He had to resolve the loose ends posed by the initial experiment. Questions abounded. Did the unnatural messenger RNA activity require UUUUUUUUUUUUUU or would UUUUUU, for example, also work? Why did some UUUUUUUUUUUUUU preparations direct protein production and others not? Could he show that the protein made in his cell extracts contained the typical chemical connections found in proteins from intact cells?[9]

The announcement of the UUUUUUUUUUUUUU experiment in Moscow vaulted Marshall into the scientific spotlight. Invitations ensued for him to come and talk about his work. Marshall declined most invitations, preferring to remain put in his lab. One invitation he did accept came from one of his scientific "heroes," Fritz Lipmann, a Nobel Laureate at the Rockefeller Institute for Medical Research in New York City. Marshall had briefly met Lipmann while still a graduate student in Michigan. When the two men met up again in Moscow, they had the opportunity for a more leisurely talk.

After his presentation in New York, Marshall asked for some important proteins that Lipmann had prepared. Marshall wanted them in order to get more details on how new protein production worked in cell extracts and to show that the proteins participated with the activity of sRNA in the making of new protein. Lipmann told Marshall that he had tried that very point but had failed.

With the samples from Lipmann in hand, Marshall returned to his lab. In one week he did all the experiments. In another week, he wrote up a paper on it. Yet, he regretted doing so. More important research awaited his attention. He had focused on how the cell extracts made new protein. Rather, he felt he should have returned to unnatural messenger RNA and the letter combinations that still remained unknown.

Competitors Emerge

Marshall's fear of competition proved prophetic. Severo Ochoa at New York University (NYU) in New York City posed an immediate threat. Ochoa was a Spanish-American doctor of medicine and a biochemist. Ochoa had received a prestigious appointment in Spain just as the Spanish Civil War erupted in 1936. After fleeing Spain and wandering for four years in Europe, Ochoa arrived in the United States. Here he began a swift rise at NYU to become the chairman of the Department of Biochemistry.

In 1955, the biochemist Marianne Grunberg-Manago worked in Ochoa's lab. She was 34 years old, having received her PhD in 1947. She discovered a protein, polynucleotide phosphorylase, that had the unusual ability to put together chemically the letters that make up the chains of RNA.[10,11]

Ochoa was 16 years older than Grunberg-Manago. Ochoa up to that time had not published a single study on RNA or DNA. Rather, he had focused on the production of energy in cells through chemical alterations of various substances. But Ochoa quickly seized on the importance of the new protein and immediately switched projects to study it. As a young researcher, and a woman, Grunberg-Manago was expected "to stand aside to let more senior colleagues take credit for group achievements, with the understanding that ... [she] will receive the same privileges later in ... her own career."[12]

In 1959, Ochoa shared the Nobel Prize in the combined category of Physiology or Medicine for discovery of this remarkable protein. Polynucleotide phosphorylase would figure heavily in Marshall's effort to unlock new letter combinations making up the genetic code. Initially thought to make RNA, researchers later discovered cells use this protein mainly to break down RNA. It mattered not. Ochoa knew about Marshall's presentation in Moscow. Now Ochoa made preparations to begin his own studies with unnatural messenger RNA. Ochoa certainly felt no adversity toward winning a second Nobel. In fact, he might have relished it.

Thus began the race to decipher how the letters making up the genetic code worked, Ochoa posed perhaps an even more formidable professional challenge to Marshall than did the RNA Tie Club. Ochoa had already an established reputation as a fierce competitor, a position that had not endeared him to others. He also kept a very tight rein on the people in his NYU lab, taking over the most promising projects for himself. As a result, his postdoctoral researchers hesitated to freely share their data with him. They put off the details for as long as possible so that they would get proper credit for their efforts. This lab culture encouraged mistakes. It prevented the much more experienced Ochoa from effectively interacting with the people in his lab during ongoing experiments.

Like Marshall, Ochoa disdained theory and focused instead on experiments and the hard data they provided. Whereas theory leaves room for improvement—theory can always be modified—hard data often proves intractable. Ochoa had also shown himself to be a prolific publisher of papers, with about 100 papers already to his credit by 1961. Marshall had published just 10. Furthermore, by having taken over the polynucleotide phosphorylase protein project, Ochoa revealed a very pragmatic approach to scientific research. Perhaps this was not unexpected given his earlier history in Europe that forced his immigration from Spain to America. Ochoa had once easily switched gears from energy to the protein, polynucleotide phosphorylase. He could do so again. With Nobel Prize in hand, Ochoa held a scientific status that cast a long shadow over Marshall.

Ochoa become interested in the use of cell extracts to make new protein in 1958, a year before Marshall even started his own studies. Ochoa first used extracts from a type of bacteria called *Alcaligenes faecalis*.[13] Despite his training as a physician, Ochoa may not have fully appreciated the human pathogenicity of this bacterium. Ochoa also used a laborious procedure to determine the amount of new protein made in his test tubes.[13] Rushing cell extracts into service, Ochoa failed to prove they produced new protein. For example, Ochoa failed to show that the new protein being made contained the expected chemical links.[13]

Peter Lengyel, an émigré to America following the Hungarian Revolution of 1956, became a graduate student with Ochoa in January1961. That summer, after Ochoa had left on vacation, Lengyel claims he independently conceived of how he might discover the genetic code. As he listened to Sydney Brenner, a member of the RNA Tie Club, lecture at the Cold Spring Harbor Laboratory on messenger RNA, Lengyel had an idea. He could use unnatural messenger RNA with cell extracts to determine the genetic code.[14] Lengyel, a mere graduate student, saw the possibilities; Brenner, a scientific icon, did not.

Marshall and Matthaei had reported in Moscow that unnatural messenger RNA could, in fact, be used in cell extracts to make new protein. Ochoa's lab now showed that the protein he had discovered, polynucleotide phosphorylase, could use two letters rather than just one to make unnatural messenger RNA. These messengers could be used like UUUUUUUUUUUUUU in cell extracts to decipher the genetic code. In addition to the messengers, Ochoa now also had a few years under his belt of using cell extracts to make new protein in test tubes. In Lengyel and Ochoa's hands, the polynucleotide phosphorylase protein had the power of a sledgehammer to smash any dreams that Marshall might enjoy in deciphering the code. Ochoa now stood on firm footing as an eminence in the cathedral of RNA research.

Like Marshall, Lengyel did not immediately recognize that he had competition. Lengyel remembers:

A friend from Rockefeller University called to let me know that there was a breakthrough in research. I remember well my first sentence to him, "Don't tell me that the genetic code was broken!" He continued, "Yes, somebody ... has found that ... [UUUUUUUUUUUUUU] ... encodes ... [the amino acid phenylalanine]. ..." I will never forget my great disappointment upon hearing that the first part of our planned project had been accomplished by somebody else. ... We decided to postpone the beginning of the experiments to consider whether and how to proceed."[15]

Lengyel initially thought to use just one letter, as Marshall and Matthaei had done, to make unnatural messenger. Lengyel later realized he could add a second letter to the mix containing the polynucleotide phosphorylase protein. The random addition of a second letter would produce an unnatural messenger RNA containing all possible three-letter combinations. If, for example, he added the letter A along with the letter U, the unnatural messenger could contain up to eight different letter combinations. He expected that such an unnatural messenger RNA could direct more than one amino acid into newly made protein. The letter combinations produced would depend on the relative amounts of U and A used. Marshall independently came up with the same idea for making unnatural messenger RNA of mixed composition. It is not uncommon for different researchers to come up with the same idea. For example, Crick had conceived of an sRNA. Someone else had discovered it without being aware of Crick's thinking.

However, the use of unnatural messenger RNA with mixed combinations of letters had two problems, not necessarily fully apparent. One was that methods to determine the exact sequence of letters in messenger RNA did not yet exist. The other was the possible contamination of one letter with a completely different letter. If the A added in the table above contained a G or a C, more three-letter combinations would result than those shown in table 8.1.

Because researchers could not determine the exact three-letter combinations directly, they had to infer them indirectly using mathematical calculations. These computations might tell them ideally what three-letter combinations could be in the unnatural messenger RNA. But the assessments could not tell them what three-letter combinations were actually there.

Marshall realized, as did Ochoa and Lengyel, that by adding different amounts of each letter, he could estimate the frequency with which one or another three-letter combination would appear in the messenger. In one example, Marshall, might use three times more of the letter U than the letter A. The total amount of letters would be $3 + 1 = 4$. The mathematical probability of obtaining the three-letter combination UUU, therefore, would be $3/4 \times 3/4 \times 3/4 = 27/4$. The mathematical probability for the three-letter combination UUA would be $3/4 \times 3/4 \times 1/4 = 9/4$. If UUU was assumed to be

Table 8.1

U	U	U
U	U	A
U	A	A
U	A	U
A	A	A
A	A	U
A	U	A
A	U	U

100 percent, UUA would be three times less (9/27) or 33 percent.[16] Although Marshall also wondered whether he could use a messenger only three to four letters long, it seemed unlikely from his experimental data.[17]

Around the middle of October 1961, Jim Watson of DNA fame invited Marshall to give a talk at MIT. People filled the large auditorium to overflowing, and latecomers had to stand in the back. Marshall had taken a day to organize his latest data, another day to make slides, and a third day to travel to Boston. These preparations robbed him of precious time in the lab. Marshall began his presentation, and during the talk Watson, as he always did, sat in the front row with the *New York Times*. During the middle of Marshall's talk, Watson unfolded the paper and vibrated it like he was angry. Marshall had heard that Watson did this during talks whenever somebody said something he didn't like or with which he disagreed. Watson's boorish behavior was unusual. Scientists usually listen attentively and critique intensively after a speaker finishes. But they do not try to interrupt the speaker this way in the middle of a presentation. Marshall, still taken aback by Watson's abject rudeness, briefly considered stopping his talk but did not do so.

Watson was not the only problem Marshall confronted that day at MIT. Lengyel, still a graduate student at NYU, had seen a notice that Marshall was to appear at MIT. Lengyel attended the talk and during the question-and-answer period that followed stood up and said he wanted to show some slides and make an announcement. He then went ahead and did so. This was another breach of scientific etiquette. One does not normally "piggyback" like this on another scientist's seminar. Lengyel had neither been invited by MIT to co-present with Marshall nor had he asked Marshall in advance whether he might do so. Rather, Lengyel should have waited to be invited to make a separate presentation at a later date.[14]

Lengyel's slides showed that the Ochoa group had used unnatural messenger RNA and had already found them directing other amino acids into new protein. Lengyel's presentation at MIT confirmed Marshall's worst fears. Marshall remembered, "Just the fact that Ochoa would send someone to give a talk after my talk was a remarkable thing. ... It was very depressing at that time because it was clear that they were way ahead of us in deciphering the code."[6]

Later, Marshall said he was used to it. Commented one observer from MIT that day, "[Someone from Ochoa's lab] ... followed Marshall around the country standing up at the end of every seminar Marshall delivered to present their ... [own work on the genetic code] ... I was shocked, and felt this to be completely unethical behavior.[18]

Marshall didn't know whether to be galvanized or paralyzed by Lengyel's announcement. He flew back to Washington feeling very unhappy. He recalled thinking, "clearly, I had to either compete with the Ochoa laboratory or stop working on the problem."[19]

Marshall had not confronted scientific competition before and, by nature, felt reticent to do so. But Lengyel's aggressive presentation at MIT dispelled any doubts Marshall may have had about Ochoa's intentions. The next month, Marshall had a chance to meet with Ochoa. Both men appeared at a meeting at the New York Academy of Medicine. Nirenberg reported his pioneering study on UUUUUUUUUUUUUU. Ochoa bested him by announcing he had deciphered 11 new letter combinations using unnatural messenger RNA made with combinations of letters rather than just one. That same afternoon, Nirenberg visited Ochoa's laboratory. But the cordial meeting failed to result in collaboration.[14] Marshall returned to Bethesda and his laboratory at NIH unsure of what to do next.

Meanwhile, in New York, Ochoa enthusiastically supported the deciphering of the genetic code that Lengyel and his associate had started. Somewhat to their dismay, Ochoa took over the project. Ochoa must have rightfully considered that the project derived from his earlier discovery (with biochemist Marianne Grunberg-Manago) of the polynucleotide phosphorylase protein.[14] Ochoa had a valid point. The NYU group used this protein to make the unnatural messenger RNA.

Ochoa had by now switched to making cell extracts from the same bacteria used by Marshall and Matthaei. Ochoa found that AAAAAAAAAAAAAA alone failed as a messenger, and when added with UUUUUUUUUUUUUU prevented it too from working as a messenger.[20] Later, researchers found that AAAAAAAAAAAAAA does, in fact, direct the production of a new protein containing just one amino acid. But the protein product did not fall out of solution as other proteins had done. Unable to find radioactive protein on their filters, the authors mistakenly assumed none had been made.

Meanwhile, Marshall wrestled with the idea, ultimately to be discarded, that one strand of the spiral staircase of DNA would make natural messenger RNA, while the other strand would make an RNA chain that would inhibit the messenger RNA. Marshall also envisioned that the dictionary of life would list only 20 three-letter combinations. Each of these letter combinations would direct the insertion of just one amino acid into protein. However, the total possible three-letter combinations that could be constructed still stood mathematically at 64. So if 20 did the actual work, what did the other 44 three-letter combinations do? Marshall predicted that another group of 20 three-letter combinations could interfere with the

20 combinations that did all the work, thereby blocking them. The remaining 24 three-letter combinations would do nothing at all.[21]

So sure was Marshall of this concept that he urged himself to publish a paper on it. Fortunately, he did not, for ultimately his data would show these ideas to be incorrect. Marshall characteristically jotted down ideas and speculation in his notebooks but refrained from sharing them in print.[22] In contrast, Ochoa might occasionally publish data without sufficient repetition or analysis and then witness it being proved incorrect.

Marshall knew that his own lack of experience rendered him far less credible than Ochoa. Therefore, Marshall had to tiptoe carefully through a minefield of research strewn with potential errors. Every experiment had to be repeated over and over again. Each published conclusion had to be carefully scrutinized. Hidden contaminants had to be ferreted out.

Marshall, for example, detected a slight addition of two other amino acids into new protein when directed by UUUUUUUUUUUUUU. Did that mean different combinations of U's in the unnatural messenger RNA could separately direct all three different amino acids into protein? Careful checking showed that the letter U he used contained the letter G as an impurity. The inclusion of the letter G in the unnatural messenger RNA resulted in new and unanticipated three-letter combinations. These new combinations accounted for why two other amino acids suddenly turned up in new protein. Checking the purity of each radioactive amino acid also showed that at least two of these also required the removal of contaminants.

Step-by-step, Marshall and Ochoa staffed their labs with MD and PhD researchers. Each new member had to be trained to make and use the cell extracts. Each had to learn how to make the unnatural messenger RNA. When experiments failed, Marshall in his lab or Ochoa at NYU had to figure out why. Contaminants played a role, of course. So too did human error from inexperienced researchers. Forging ahead, the Ochoa group made unnatural messenger RNA with different letter combinations and different proportions.[14] Lengyel recalled, "Watching the ... [instrument that counted radioactivity] ... with Dr. Ochoa and ... and witnessing that .... [the two unnatural messengers] ... promote[d] the uptake of other particular amino acids ... were among the greatest joys of my scientific career.[23]

Like Marshall, the Ochoa group also remained unclear about exactly how unnatural messenger RNA worked. When speculation replaced hard experimental data, errors became inescapable. A paper by Ochoa on the function of unnatural messenger RNAs containing three-letter combinations of U and C provided a case in point. Unnatural messenger RNA made from a combination of the letters U and C in a 5:1 proportion worked well.

When they reversed the letter proportions of U and C as 1: 5, the unnatural messenger RNA made seemed almost ineffective.[20]

The authors speculated, later shown to be incorrect, on a reason for this difference. They thought that three-letter combinations that coded for amino acids in unnatural messenger RNA required stretches of the letter U in between to hold them together. When unnatural messenger RNA lacked this structure, they directed the linking together of only short chains of amino acids. These small chains would not fall out of solution and so would go undetected. Thus, the unnatural messenger RNA made with the 5:1 proportions had the right structure. The unnatural messenger made with 1:5 proportions did not and so had coding gaps that led to the smaller chains.

Just as Marshall felt competitive pressure from Ochoa, Lengyel at NYU remained concerned about Marshall as well. Neither group knew the precise order of three-letter combinations in the unnatural messenger RNA they made. Their mathematical calculations gave theoretical, not actual, compositions. For one unnatural messenger RNA made by Ochoa, the computed three-letter combinations might be UAC, UCA, ACU, AUC, CUA or CAU.[24] Eventually, the correct three-letter combinations from later experiments turned out to be CAU and CAC. Yet the three-letter combination CAC went unaccounted for in their paper. Similarly, three-letter combinations for two other amino acids would later prove to also be wrong in papers published by the NYU group.

In the *Bulletin of the New York Academy of Medicine*, Ochoa addressed the direction in which the polynucleotide phosphorylase protein made unnatural messenger RNA. Direction of production was important in trying to match the correct order of amino acids in protein to the order of the three-letter combinations in the messenger RNA.

Ochoa declared that making the messenger RNA proceeded from right to left. He opined that the production of protein went from left to right.[25] Ochoa made a mistake, because later results showed that production of the messenger RNA went from left to right as shown below and the production of protein went the opposite way.

5' pApUpUpUpUpUpUpUpUpUpUplJ••••••••••pUpUpU 3'

(COOH) amino acid-amino acid-amino acid•••••••••••amino acid (NH₂)

Thus, in the push for priority, rapid publication sometimes interfered with the rigorous testing demanded by these difficult experiments. In the final analysis, such mistakes proved costly to the Ochoa group. Marshall remained a virtual unknown before he announced the results of the

UUUUUUUUUUUUUU experiment. Forced by inclination, inexperience, and potential embarrassment to be more conservative, Marshall knew his data had to be absolutely correct.

In the long run, Ochoa and Lengyel appeared to have outraced Marshall to decipher the functions of the various three-letter combinations. In reality, Ochoa and Lengyel ended up disqualified. They had violated a cardinal principle of scientific research. Science is built fact upon fact. There is no room for unreliable results. The publication mistakes made by the NYU group cast doubt on their credibility. Judgment of their work proved costly to them. Somehow, Marshall dodged the criticisms hurled at Ochoa. In the end, Marshall emerged somewhat unscathed.

At the time, however, the future likelihood for either Marshall or Ochoa's success looked dim. The use of unnatural messenger RNA with its mixtures of three-letter combinations was leading nowhere. Neither man could figure out the exact order of the three-letter combinations in each messenger RNA. Either one or the other would have to find an alternative approach. Otherwise, the alphabet of life would remain a soupy mess for understanding the chemical basis of heredity.

9 Nirvana

In 1961, Marshall and Matthaei published their UUUUUUUUUUUUUU experiment. Fame came to them as a result. At the end of the year, the editors of *Scientific American* solicited articles from both Crick and Marshall. Yet, they planned to publish Crick's article first. Crick felt he had to explain that the basic discovery of Marshall and Matthaei had come *before* his results with Brenner from the virus studies that suggested, but did not prove, a three-letter combination for the code.[1]

On the other side of the Atlantic, on December 31, 1961, the *Observer's* science correspondent, quipped:

A major advance in unraveling the secrets of life appears imminent. A paper published in *Nature* yesterday, by four Cambridge scientists, suggests that the "genetic code" is about to be cracked. ... [They] believe they have established what type of code is involved. This, as all cryptographers know, is the most important step towards cracking any code. ... This work is developing at such a pace that the layman cannot be expected to keep up."[1]

The *Observer* referred to the Crick, Brenner, and associates paper on the general nature of the genetic code for proteins. Marshall and Matthaei's discovery of the first actual code word got mentioned, but almost as an afterthought.

By the summer of 1962, Ochoa's actions signaled his intention to battle Marshall. His resumé listed winner of the Nobel Prize, recipient of honorary degrees, and chair of the Department of Biochemistry at NYU. Marshall could only claim being a low-level staff scientist at a federal government laboratory. Measuring his adversary, Ochoa saw little reason to step aside from his research on the code. Certainly, Marshall and Matthaei had deciphered the first code word in the dictionary of life. But the genetic vocabulary likely consisted of 63 other code words. Ochoa was determined to find the rest of them.

As the department chair at NYU, Ochoa also wielded influence and power. Wasting no time, he added fresh recruits to his lab staff. One brought financial support as a fellow of the Jane Coffin Childs Fund for Medical Research and another came with financial support as an international fellow of the National Institutes of Health, U.S. Public Health Service. The group wasted no time in preparing unnatural messenger RNA, testing each one in cell extracts, and determining which amino acids responded to the unnatural message RNA by showing up in new protein.

But other battles of far greater consequence thundered and roared in far-off Vietnam. The Vietnam War also needed recruits. Those recruits came as a result of the Selective Service Act of 1948 that required all men, ages 18 to 26, to register for the draft. The Act also created the "Doctor Draft" aimed at inducting health professionals into military service. Unless otherwise exempted or deferred, doctors could be called for up to 21 months of active duty and five years of reserve duty service. Marshall's medical history and his age now exempted him from the draft but not from a significant advantage the draft would hand him. Marshall would share a Nobel Prize, in part, as an unintended consequence of the Vietnam War.

Highly trained and extraordinarily intelligent, some doctors would not have to go immediately off to war. But for a few even more select others, still another pathway out of the Vietnam quagmire beckoned. In a highly competitive program, a limited number of top-notch doctors could hook up with the U.S. Public Health Service. These self-described "Yellow Berets" took their moniker from the heroic United States Army Special Forces termed the "Green Berets."[2] For those doctors lucky enough to traverse this public health route, their journey could ultimately bring them to the doorstep of NIH. There, Marshall among others awaited, while contending with Ochoa, the RNA Tie Club, and others in the battle to decipher the genetic code.

Competition for placement as research associates in the public health service proved extremely arduous. In July 1963, for example, NIH accepted only 53 doctors out of 1,464 applicants for duty.[2] Donald S. Frederickson, a former director of NIH, and himself many years earlier a participant in the program, said, "The best, the absolute cream, the 'Tiffanys,' all applied. Each Institute would do their damnedest to get what they considered the best."[2] When Frederickson went through the current applications, he realized that very few had done any research. Nevertheless, he told an associate, if he were applying for the program now, he would never be accepted given the very high quality of the current applicants.[2]

In the meantime, Marshall could claim to have definitively discovered only two code words in the genetic dictionary. Consequently, the absence of further discoveries would undermine the global acclaim he had just received in Moscow. Judith Levin, one of the few women with a doctoral degree to later join Marshall's lab, still remembers those early days. What astounded Levin and so many other scientists was that because of Marshall, "the genetic code was susceptible to simple biochemical analysis. It was ... really a defining moment in the history of science."[3]

Wanting to hedge their bets, the directors of NIH steered a steady stream of research associates to Marshall's laboratory. One NIH staff member recalls, "We all knew each other. ... [We knew] ... that Marshall ... [was]... competing with Ochoa, and ... [that] ... we ought to help him because it would be good for NIH ... Bob [Martin] was that kind of guy and he just ... [dove] ... in and spent quite a fair amount of time just helping Marshall."[4]

Early on, Martin saw the potential of Marshall's research for resolving the genetic code. Martin modestly recalls, "It was clearly the most exciting problem around, and you know, I didn't take that much time to do it. ... I felt sorry for ... [Marshall] ... that Ochoa was gonna scoop him ... and God, what could be a more exciting problem than that?"[5]

Martin recalled, "We at NIH were terribly angry with Ochoa and his colleagues for jumping in on Marshall and ... [Matthaei's] ... discovery. But of course, they too were working on protein synthesis at the time. ... Ochoa's director of operations, says they had planned those experiments before hearing of Marshall's work. I am sure he is right."[6]

With staff from NIH prepared to take time from their own research to help him, Marshall felt elated. "Given the choice," he said, "I would much prefer to collaborate with people, not to compete, although I found that I liked to compete too. I never realized this until I was actually forced into this situation with Ochoa."[7]

Yet, others at NIH did not share Martin's enthusiasm for Marshall. Rather, they took a more nuanced view of him. "None of the rest of us thought Marshall was somebody who—if we had to predict ... could do great things—I don't think anybody would've picked Marshall."[4] Another remembered, "[Tomkins] ... started telling me about this guy Nirenberg and the great things he was doing. But somehow they always fizzled up; he had great ideas, but they didn't get anywhere. And so then ... [Tomkins] ... told me one day about Marshall's work with the genetic code and I thought, 'Ugh, here we go again.'"[8]

The experiment Marshall reported on in Moscow signaled not an end to research on the genetic code but a beginning. Marshall had used the one unnatural messenger RNA, UUUUUUUUUUUUUU, that worked best. GGGGGGGGGGGGGGG would not have, for it twists on itself, preventing function as a messenger. The use of AAAAAAAAAAAAAA would produce a protein consisting of just one amino acid. But the product would initially escape detection because it would not fall out of solution. If it did not fall out of solution, the filter would contain no radioactivity. The unnatural messenger RNA CCCCCCCCCCCCCC barely functioned, for reasons unknown.[9] Today we understand the technical basis of these problems, but at the time, they led Marshall and others astray, thinking that perhaps all messenger RNA had to contain the letter U. The final results would prove that messengers did not necessarily need any letters of U.[9] Still the exact number of letters spelling out a code word remained unclear.

Moving On to Find Answers

Like Ochoa, Marshall now sought to make unnatural messenger RNA containing two or more letter combinations. The number of possible letter combinations depended on how much of each letter Marshall used to make the messenger RNA. More than one amino acid was expected to respond to such a messenger RNA. But figuring out which combination of letters gave rise to which amino acids in the proteins proved more difficult.[10] Marshall soon added another member besides Matthaei to his laboratory—Oliver Jones. Jones had initially wanted nothing more than to be an outstanding physician. That is, until he discovered Watson and Crick's seminal paper on the structure of DNA. Later, awarded a research associate position at NIH, Jones found his way to Gordon Tomkins. He recalled, "I listed Gordon first and he said, 'Bill, I just don't have any openings, I'm full. But there's a guy down the hall in my group by the name of Marshall Nirenberg, and he's doing some pretty interesting research. Maybe you ought to go talk to him,' and so that's how it came about."[11]

The variable results with each new unnatural messenger RNA led Marshall to conclude that in many cases, only the first two letters of each letter combination were fixed. If the third letter were a U, it might behave as if it were a G, C, or perhaps even an A.[12] In other cases, the letter C in the third position could act like the letter U; the letter A like the letter G.[13] What caused this variability remained unclear.

Marshall thought it might have to do with how the straight linear chain of letters in the messenger RNA could twist and turn on itself. The contortions could affect how sRNA, an essential component of his extracts, interacted with the messenger RNA.[14] Yet, at the same time, Marshall considered these ideas of messenger RNA gymnastics speculative and not ready for discussion.[15] But if correct, the results implied that the combination of letters coding for each amino acid in the messenger RNA consisted of just two letters. A genetic code consisting of only two letters rather than three had already been proposed by others.[16] But clear evidence for such a code remained thin at best.

Norma Zabriskie Heaton, who worked with Marshall for 40 years as a technician, remembered that "the lab work was intensive, exciting, and downright fun. But it could also be frustrating, stressful and tedious. Marshall wrote out the protocols to follow and left them on the lab bench," said Zabriskie Heaton. His handwriting could be challenging to decipher, but, like learning a foreign language, it became easier with time. He told me it was because he was a natural lefty, forced to learn to write with his right hand."[17]

Zabriskie Heaton noted, "Marshall was modest, soft-spoken and kind. He was a true gentleman, and it was his nature to be generous with praise. He was very creative and had so many ideas—he liked to try them out with fast little experiments just to see where they might lead—he called them "quickies."[17]

In the lab, Marshall still worried about the cell extracts "pooping" out of energy. He felt that so many things could go wrong: a fall in the salt concentration, clogging of the ribosomes where proteins got made, using up of essential ingredients, or even inhibition by small pieces of degraded messenger RNA.[18] In addition, many questions about the initial experiment still abounded. Why, for example, could a messenger RNA like UUUUUUUUUUUUUU also direct two other amino acids into protein? Potential culprits included contaminants of either the chemical letter used to make the messenger RNA, the amino acids, or both. Marshall and Matthaei grew nervous over these discrepancies.

The abundance of contaminants drove Marshall batty. As a result, Marshall demanded rigorous attention to the purity of all products being used, particularly if they came from outside sources. Marshall passed these tenets on to the research associates and others whom he trained. Sidney Pestka, a research associate, for example, took Marshall's training to heart. When Pestka eventually set up his own laboratory at NIH, he invited Robert Gallo to join him. Gallo would later become famous for his role in the discovery of viruses that cause AIDS and cancer.

"If anybody was rigorous," says Gallo, "it was ... [Pestka]. ... So I feel like I worked with Marshall because ... [Pestka] ... would always go back on that. When he was pretty tough with me, he'd say, 'Well, Marshall would demand [it].' He always used Marshall [as the standard]. ... [Pestka] almost killed me. … He didn't believe [in] anything that he got commercially. … Sidney used to say, 'How do you know histidine … [an amino acid] … is histidine, how do you know leucine … [another amino acid] … is leucine?' And I'd say, 'Okay.' He wanted me to do the electrophoresis, you know that high voltage stuff … [to confirm purity] … and after almost getting killed, I said 'Sidney, let's think about this together. How do you know water is water?'"[19]

In the afterglow of his presentation in Moscow, Marshall's mind teemed with questions, lonely for want of answers. Could UUUUUUUUUUUUUU work as a single chain or did it have to be a double chain like the spiral staircase of DNA? When he tested other unnatural messenger RNA as both single and double chains, only the single forms worked. Then he wondered how much more could he shorten UUUUUUUUUUUUUU and still get it to work? Puzzling over this last question would enable Marshall to compile virtually the complete dictionary of the genetic code.[20]

Yet, each question he answered led to two new ones. This is typical of laboratory research in science. Was each chain of UUUUUUUUUUUUUU used repeatedly by the cell extract or just once?[20,21] How could he best optimize his cell extracts and keep them in top shape?[22] How could he be certain that what went on in his cell extracts resembled what went on in intact cells?[23]

Marshall had no textbook to which he could turn for answers. Rather, *he* would potentially write the dictionary on the genetic code. But it would take years of experiments to fill up the pages laying out the letters of the code. UUUUUUUUUUUUUU has two ends. The instructions to begin making protein presumably starts from one end. But which end? The right or the left? Marshall figured he could test the effects of damaging one end. If protein production began with the letter combinations at that end of the chain, the production of protein would stop.[21] If production continued, it must have started from the opposite end.

Marshall struggled to decipher how the letters making up the code worked together. Meanwhile, in France, François Jacob and Jacques Monod studied how intact cells made information in their DNA available. Enamored with Jacob and Monod's ideas, Marshall tried to fit his data to theirs. He thought that messenger RNA copied from one side of the spiral staircase of DNA could start production of protein. Messenger RNA copied from the other side of the DNA staircase could stop it. Marshall also felt that messenger RNA might break down into smaller pieces during the making of protein. The fragments could perhaps block further protein production. He wondered how the inducers of protein production identified by Jacob and Monod worked? He thought they might be "plumbers" that unclogged ribosomes, where proteins got made. In this way, the ribosomes could be reused.[24] In these speculative ideas, Marshall was largely incorrect. But Marshall's idea of two copies of RNA acting in opposition to one another was basically correct. Decades later, others would use one form of RNA to block messenger RNA and so help cure disease.

Both Marshall and members of the RNA Tie Club speculated on how the arrangement of letters in messenger RNA directed the order of amino acids in proteins. Crick believed each letter combination for an amino acid had to be separated from the next combination by a sort of chemical comma. Crick declared, "All ... [comma-less] ... codes are unlikely, not only because of the genetic evidence but also because of the detailed results from the ... [cell extracts]."[25] Marshall disagreed. The letter combinations, he believed, stood tightly against each other in messenger RNA with nothing separating one from the next.[26] Marshall thought that some amino acids might respond to more than one combination of letters. He also speculated that a basic combination of at least three letters directed the insertion of each amino acid into protein. Each three-letter unit would be lined up with the next thereby forming a continuous single chain of messenger RNA. In these ideas, his later data would show him to be correct.

Marshall toyed with the idea that some letter combinations might have no function at all. Such combinations would not code for *any* amino acid. Alternatively, every letter combination might have a function. If so, that would increase the likelihood that some amino acids could respond to more than one combination of letters. If this latter prediction proved true, Marshall realized, it ruled out the proposal Gamow made to the RNA Tie Club.[26] Gamow's proposal could accommodate 20 different letter combinations, but no more than that.

Clearly, with so many questions yet unanswered, Marshall needed all the help he could get. Chance meetings in the NIH parking lot with Bob Gallo led Marshall to invite him to join the work on the genetic code. Initially accepting the offer, Gallo later reneged. "Probably down deep, there was a major factor of insecurity that I ... [was] ... really not ready. I knew some enzymology, but what the hell did I really know about ... [sRNA] ... and about the code and about differentiation?"[19] Instead, Gallo ended up with Pestka, who had by then graduated from Marshall's lab to one of his own.

Going to the Greats

Marshall saw the limits of making unnatural messenger RNA with different combinations of letters. He had consequently based all of his ideas up to now on faulty data.[27] Marshall realized he knew little about the chemistry of linking letters together. He needed help. This chemistry required specialized training. Marshall's previous education, training, and experience had left him unprepared. So he sought the advice of the world's three greatest biological chemists in this field: Leon Heppel, Gobind Khorana, and Alexander Todd.

Gobind Khorana had been a nomadic scientist, moving about from one country to another. Born in what is now East Pakistan, he received his degree in England, then spent time in Switzerland, migrated to Canada, and by 1962 came to the United States. There he joined the University of Wisconsin. Khorana focused on making in the laboratory short single chains of DNA. He could control and know the exact arrangement of letters in the chain. Then, with a special protein, he copied the letters from DNA into messenger RNA. He added each unnatural messenger RNA to cell extracts as Marshall and Ochoa did. Khorana could then match the exact arrangement of letters in the unnatural messenger RNA with the exact order of amino acids in the protein made in response. Thus, Khorana avoided guessing at which letter combinations in the unnatural messenger RNA specified which amino acids. Marshall's and Ochoa's use simply of different letter combinations to make unnatural messenger RNA gave ambiguous results.

Todd had worked out exactly how the letters of DNA linked one to the next. His impressive body of chemical triumphs led to his being knighted in 1954, and raised to the peerage eight years later. He received the title of Baron Todd of Trumpington.

However, Marshall disliked the cross-country and cross-oceanic distance from Khorana and Todd, respectively. Therefore, Marshall turned to someone closer: Leon Heppel at NIH proved more to his liking. Heppel, who had once collaborated with Ochoa, like others at NIH, wanted to help Marshall. But unlike the others, Heppel may have been particularly motivated. Says Charles O'Neal, who later joined Marshall, "I think the association with Heppel was definitely an advantage ... [for Marshall] ... Now this is pure rumor, pure guestimate on my part. I think Heppel was somewhat irritated at Ochoa ... [for] ... not giving him some credit on the polynucleotide phosphorylase story ... [that earned Ochoa the Nobel Prize]."[28]

O'Neal recalled, "[At a meeting], I was standing behind ... [Ochoa] ... on an escalator. He ... [was] ... discussing the rumor that Marshall had finally cracked the rest of the code, and I overheard him say, 'Well, we don't know what they have, and we'll have to wait till tomorrow and see' ... I just kept my mouth shut."[28]

Says Gary Felsenfeld who later met with Ochoa, " I remember the stories ... of the outrage on the part of the NIH community that here this guy [Ochoa] who was already a Nobel Laureate felt that he had to compete with a young guy who was making a great discovery. And ... [Ochoa] ... was expressing ... his judgment, if I understood what he was saying ... that he wished he hadn't done it."[29]

Perhaps Ochoa felt embarrassed for having won the Nobel Prize for a protein whose function later turned out to be different than expected. This might have motivated him to seek a second award.

Heppel helped Marshall defend his discovery against Ochoa's grasp. Heppel's brilliance as a chemist remained undimmed by his idiosyncratic nature. His fastidiousness in the laboratory extended to the cleanliness of doorknobs that he touched, paper towels, and even his own hands.[5] In the fall, for example, on the 9th floor at NIH, "he'd come running down the hall to all the labs. He'd go, 'Okay everybody, out of the lab, out of the lab,' and we'd follow him, you know the whole 50 people or something ... down and around the corner ... and look out ... at the colors of the leaves changing and he'd say, 'See isn't that beautiful? Okay, now get back to work.'"[5]

But he had another side as well. "Leon Heppel was a remarkable person," says Jones. "[Heppel was] extremely shy. And if I said Marshall was meticulous, Heinrich [Matthaei] was meticulous, Leon Heppel was meticulous to the 10th power. It's just unbelievable, but he was doing work ... where this was an absolute requirement."[11]

Other memories of Heppel's eccentricities abound. Jones recalls that Heppel remained very active in the lab. He wanted things done a certain way, no matter who you were. Once, Khorana, a future Nobel Laureate, visited. Heppel did not like how Khorana was doing something and slapped Khorana's hands. Heppel meant to correct Khorana's technique, not humiliate him.[11]

About Heppel, Gary Felsenfeld, another researcher at NIH, recalls, "I remember very well ... [Heppel] ... used to bring his family with him on Sunday. And if you went into this lab on a Sunday, you'd see him on the bench and his kids on the floor reading comics. His family was in the lab while he worked. .... [In addition], Heppel wanted to see who could work the fastest, and somebody got the idea to pour his breakfast cereal into his jacket pocket so he could eat while working. These were serious people."[29]

Marshall's reaching out to Heppel and Khorana revealed a sense of confidence in the 34-year-old man. After years of wandering through his career, sky-high opportunity had at last beckoned. It was no time to be solitary, shy, or inhibited. "Go into organic synthesis seriously," Marshall jotted in his notebook. "Learn all techniques. Become expert in literature. Visit Khorana and/or Todd. ... Get Heppel to give lectures on Khorana, Todd. ... Big job but necessary. Need expert organic chemist." [30]

Marshall admitted he needed to confirm the order of letters in unnatural messenger RNA. He thought there were two ways to do this. Chemical addition was one: a step-by-step linking of one letter to the next. The use of a special protein was the other: a biological "stitching" together of the letters.[31] When Brian Clark joined his lab, Marshall had the man to handle the chemical syntheses.

Clark learned of the opportunity with Marshall through friends. Before he could accept, however, the Massachusetts Institute of Technology had to release him from his three-year contract. Like researchers at NIH, those at MIT also supported Marshall's efforts and so sent Clark forth. Clark arrived in 1962 along with two other research associates Philip Leder and Sidney Pestka. They came just as three others were leaving Marshall's lab. Says Clark, "Marshall realized that the main competition would not be NYU ... [and Ochoa] ... but Madison [Wisconsin] ... in the form of Gobind Khorana's group that had taken over from Cambridge University as the chief ... [makers] ... of ... [unnatural messenger RNA]."[32]

Marshall feared that his taste of success would soon be swallowed up by the competition. He needed as much help as possible. When he had three people, he found he needed six.[33] He also needed to replace people after they completed their appointments in his lab. The need for more people brought with it the need for more space.[34] Nirenberg figured that four shared laboratory modules might be enough.[35]

Zabriskie Heaton recalled, "The labs were all crowded—we didn't work side by side—it was elbow to elbow. It was so busy that Theresa [Caryk, another technician] labeled ... [one of our bottles of chemicals] ... in Ukrainian so that it didn't wander off. Marshall had a tiny office in the back part of our single module lab just wide enough for his desk, two chairs and a file cabinet, and you usually had to clear off a chair in order to sit down."[17]

But Marshall's dream of chasing down the genetic code was becoming a nightmare. The National Institute of Arthritis, Metabolism and Digestive Diseases at NIH, in which Marshall worked, either could not or would not support further expansion of his group. Completely absorbed in his research, Marshall had little time and, perhaps, less inclination, to leave NIH. Marshall realized that the resources potentially available at NIH easily outstripped anything he could accrue at a university. Rather than having it handed to him at NIH, he would be forced to apply for grant support at a university. Marshall explained, "I would never have been awarded a grant to do the work because I had no experience in the field. … It was such far-out work, and it was in '58 such a highly competitive field, that nobody would have given me a grant to do it."[7]

Marshall's wife Perola played a key role in Marshall's latest dilemma. Marshall risked everything by announcing he was leaving NIH. Perola, trained as a biochemist, now also worked at NIH for Sidney Udenfriend, another staff member. Udenfriend held a position in the National Heart Institute at NIH. Previously, as a graduate student, he had begun his PhD program at NYU under future Nobel Laureate Severo Ochoa. When Ochoa left after one year, to go to another department at NYU, Udenfriend had to scramble to find a new thesis advisor. A few years after graduating, Udenfriend received an invitation to join NIH, where he met up with Perola. Prior to accepting the position at NIH, Udenfriend had been advised to reject it. "If you join a little known government laboratory," he was told, "this will be the end of your scientific career!"[36] It was anything but the end.

Perola asked Udenfriend for time off to go with Marshall to the University of Michigan. Michigan had offered Marshall an appointment as assistant professor of human genetics. However, for some reason, the appointment seemed tentative, for it only ran from January to June, with a salary of $12,000.[37] Herbert Weissbach, who worked with Udenfriend, said, "[Udenfriend] … didn't want to lose Perola. I don't think he was that interested in Marshall. … So he called us all in and said, 'Listen, if we all cut our space in half … we'll have enough space for Marshall.' We said, 'Fine, no problem.'" Udenfriend asked the research director of the Heart Institute to accommodate the under-appreciated Marshall, and he moved with his staff into Udenfriend's lab.[38]

By September 1962, Marshall faced mounting pressure as his research project burgeoned. He noted, "[I] am not part of [a] good group like [a] department. No one [physically] close to talk to," although, he noted "[the] telephone is perfect for questions."[39] Marshall had no intention of waiting three to five years for the perfect set-up. Instead, he wanted the large group the project called for now. He estimated he would need space for 20 people. Even by placing two to three people at each laboratory bench, he would still need nine modules. He also wanted rooms for a library, instruments, large-scale preparation of biological components ranging from bacterial cells to ribosomes, and office space. Additional personnel would have to include a dishwasher, preparation manager, lab manager, and, two technicians.

His ideal staff would consist of about six superb PhD graduates to work on various aspects of his research projects. Each PhD graduate would have a doctor inexperienced in research—one of the research associates—to train.

He didn't want to supervise the PhD graduates in minute detail. Rather, he would assign each one to do part or all of a research project in his lab and expect them to function independently. He had little time to spend thinking about their research projects.[40]

He would leave the PhD graduates alone but arrange to see them once a week for a conference. If they had sufficient experience, he would let them draft the papers for publication and would then review the semifinal drafts.[41] As far as he was concerned, he once again urged himself to focus attention on his own work. He wanted as much free time as possible to do this, particularly for new work. This arrangement, he felt, was necessary so that if a new development occurred in his lab, he could switch gears and get right on it.

All of this was wishful thinking. In reality, Marshall would find even less time to interact with his staff than he ever imagined. Even with a large group to help him, Marshall was beset with doubts and quandaries. The experiments on the three-letter combinations for particular amino acids failed to give consistent results even when checked two or three times.[42] Each new batch of cell extracts and the same unnatural messenger RNA produced variations in the production of proteins. Despite painstaking attention to detail, Marshall failed to find the reason for these differences. Almost the entire dictionary of the three-letter combinations remained to be deciphered. The experimental inconsistencies grew intolerable.

Marshall's Team Assembles

By September 1962, the group had expanded to nine people. Only about five years past his own graduation from Michigan, Marshall now had a bevy of young, often inexperienced research associates to direct. How could he manage all this? Marshall decided to give each member of his lab an independent problem to work on individually. One person, for example, would research which direction the cell extracts read the messenger RNA. Another would work on alternative ways to use a special protein to make the unnatural messenger RNA. Marshall himself would work on yet a different problem.[43]

Philip Leder came to Marshall's lab sometime after failing to follow his own father's advice. Leder declined the appointment he received to the U.S. Naval Academy despite his father's protestations. Instead, Leder opted for Harvard University. Between his second and third year of college, he thought he would be a playground supervisor in the summer. Instead, he ended up in a lab at NIH. Leder described that summer as "a wonderful experience, I enjoyed it enormously. I couldn't believe that people did this sort of thing and, and could make a living out of it."[44] After going on to Harvard Medical School, Leder completed his residency at the University of Minnesota before joining Marshall's lab. Later, he would become the founder of the Department of Genetics at Harvard Medical School.

Recalled Leder, "I knew nothing when I came to ... [Marshall's] ... lab ... I had a good course in organic chemistry but no biochemistry and no technique, so I felt that ... [it would] ... be much better to listen to ... the suggestions that ... [Marshall] ... might make and, and accept them, pending the time, when I would feel that I can be independent, in both choice of project and its execution."[44]

Sidney Pestka arrived at Marshall's lab via Princeton University and the University of Pennsylvania School of Medicine. Leder and Petska worked together, albeit sometimes uneasily. They took turns being responsible for preparing the ribosomes from the cell extracts. Each was a perfectionist in his own way. Pestka managed to "squeeze" more ribosomes out of each extract than did Leder.[44]

Despite the help of people like Leder and Pestka, Marshall felt pressured, He chafed at what he perceived as the slow progress of work each day. He sensed that his best defense against Ochoa, the RNA Tie Club, and Khorana rested on making rapid progress in deciphering the code. Clearly, he needed to speed things up. New technical developments played a key role. One involved an invention by Leder, subsequently patented, of simultaneously filtering at one time the contents of 45 test tubes rather than one at a time. Radioactive protein newly made by a cell extract stuck to the filter while other material passed through. The amount of radioactivity counted on the filter measured the extent of protein production.

Yet, Leder said, despite the growing pressure, Marshall remained "soft spoken." He would patiently listen to a younger colleague and give serious thought to his or her question or idea, no matter how off-beat. Colleagues were invariably greeted by a cheery, "So what's new?" And he really wanted to hear what was going on in the lab. Science was clearly his all-consuming passion. Conversations with him were always stimulating. He retained that gleeful enthusiasm he exhibited as a teenager, catching snakes in a Florida swamp."[45]

Once again, Marshall felt the need to urge himself onward. "Let [the] section work for me, not me work for section. Maintain individual research. Give others responsibility. Delegate responsibility."[46] He further noted, "Many ideas come only from research and are suggested by reading and thinking about only [a] few papers. Must do some lab work and ... [I] ...

must keep in absolute and complete touch with 1 piece of research. ... New good ideas [should] go to new people coming in. Work with about 5 people—trained biochem[ists]. Each has [an] independent project related to 1 or 2 central [ideas]. Define project. Talk about problems, etc. Do not care if [the] project does not work out. [I] ... can give each trained person an untrained person to teach."[46]

Marshall felt responsible for creating an exciting, intellectual environment for the young people flocking to his lab. However, he himself needed his personal space. He planned to make his personal lab and office off limits for three-fourths of each day. He wanted to keep his time free for meditation, thinking, and reading. His day involved working late and then sleeping late. He reminded himself: "Don't be [a] perfectionist. Let people make their own mistakes. Only care that the work that you, yourself are doing gets done. Push that [work] hard. Work predominantly on far-out problems. Push this philosophy to colleagues. Don't look for quantity publications—quality instead. Imagination. Originality. Superb craftsmanship. Under no circumstances be pushed into publishing sloppy work."[46]

Now that Marshall had partially beaten a pathway to the code, other labs began to follow suit. Marshall spent considerable time critically reading their papers, seeking to make sense of their work and his. Sometimes these papers helped; sometimes they did not. Marshall spent much time trying to reconcile his data with theirs. His notebooks detail struggles to make sense of these new papers.

Marshall also realized he needed a new way to solve how the messenger RNA placed amino acids in the correct order in each protein. Two objectives underscored his redesigned approach. How to resolve the smallest number of letters that made up a code word was one. The other involved adding three different letters to the back end of UUUUUUUUUUUUUU. The redesigned messenger would make a protein containing just one amino acid but add at the very end a second amino acid. The exact order of the three letters at the end would reveal the combination of letters that led to that very last amino acid.[47]

Zabriskie Heaton experienced Marshall as "very focused and demanding. He had a meticulous and painstaking approach to data analysis. ... When you discussed your results with him, he expected you to know your experiments inside and out, backward and forward. No detail was overlooked or insignificant to him. ... You had better know which solutions you used, who made them, when they were made, how they were made and the ... [manufacturer's] ... lot number of every ... [chemical]."[17]

Yet, for Marshall at this juncture, hope alternated with despair. "[I'm] very stuck at this point on the code and [am] going around in circles," he wrote.[48] He could not yet foresee that his salvation lay with the size of the message. So he clung to his earlier idea of inducing production of a protein and analyzing its messenger RNA. Marshall worked with as many as five different bacteria and methods of inducing new production of protein. Each bacterial cell and induction scheme led to the production of a different new protein.[49] He still failed to notice for each experiment the lack of needed methods to analyze both the order of amino acids in the proteins and the arrangement of letters in the messenger RNA.

Yet, variable results continued to plague the experiments with cell extracts and unnatural messenger RNA. Therefore, Marshall cautiously thought the data qualitatively, but not quantitatively, valid. At this point, he knew only that some amino acids responded to multiple letter combinations, that the letter U was not always required, and that at least two letters were required to direct each amino acid. Marshall still did not know if three-letter combinations constituted one coding unit.[50] For him, this remained a puzzle.

However, members of the RNA Tie Club, particularly Crick, had no such concerns. They touted a genetic code consisting of three letters despite the absence of hard data to support it. In his Nobel Lecture in 1962, Crick emphasized the term "triplet" to describe the three-letter size of the code no fewer than 37 times.[25]

How, Marshall wondered, were multiple letter combinations for certain amino acids related? He envisioned a slippage of some sort with the third letter A, for example, matching with the letter C instead of the usual letter U. In any case, the slippage action was *nonrandom*, he emphasized.[51] The idea of slippage—later to be christened "wobble"—helped clarify the idea that the code consisted of three letters, not two. However, whereas the first two letters were fixed, the third letter gave added flexibility. Thus, a standard 3-letter combination came to dominate Marshall's thinking.

Marshall now had so much going on in his laboratory, and a larger group to carry out the work. But he felt it increasingly difficult to concentrate. "Interruptions," he noted, "[are] bad. Better if I go see [the] secretary or call when free. [I] must work quietly. If interrupted, tell [people I'm busy. .... [Take] appointments ... only after 4:30. Concentrate on 1 thing. No distractions"[52]

But a big change was about to take place. On a Saturday night, undated but just before Thanksgiving 1963, Marshall prophetically wrote in his notebook, "[sRNA] ... goes to ribosome in presence of m[essenger] RNA.

Will ... [just a 3-letter combination] ... substitute for ... [an entire] ....
m[essenger]RNA? Could use this technique to get code word sequence."[53]
This was just one of the countless ideas that passed through his notebooks.
But this idea unlike the others would matter far more. Marshall's use of just
a 3-letter messenger would be the highway he would ride to the project's
successful completion. Even so, he would have to avoid many experimental
"potholes" along the way.

Marshall spent Thanksgiving Day, 1963, thinking about how to test this
new idea. Should the sRNA be added, for example, before or after the three-
letter combination?[54] He pondered over the details for about a month.
Then Marshall asked Leder to do the experiment. Marshall provided details
of how various steps were to be done. The filters to be used, how the ribosomes should be washed, the order of addition of each critical component
from the cell extracts.[55] This experiment would finally lead Marshall out of
the intellectual wilderness in which he was floundering. He would finally
discover both the exact number of letters and the letter combinations
needed for each amino acid.

By April 1964, this crucial insight had pushed the project back on track.
With data in hand, Leder remembers, "I walked into his little office. I was
scarcely able to contain myself, and I asked him how long he thought ...
[a message] ... had to be to get recognition? I don't know whether he said
it because he believed it or whether he said it because he was afraid to be
overly optimistic or enthusiastic, but he said, oh, I don't remember exactly,
but some number bigger than six, maybe around nine or ten ... [letters].
So I think I put it to him, 'Would you believe six, would you believe five,
would you believe *three*' or something like that. And he nearly jumped out
of his skin."[56]

Leder had found that a particular sRNA bearing a specific radioactive
amino acid could be bound to a ribosome by just a three-letter messenger.
Each sRNA has a three-letter combination that has to match in a certain
way to a three-letter combination in the messenger RNA. For each amino
acid, there is a special sRNA with a different three-letter combination to
match to the messenger RNA.

If the sRNA recognized the three-letter combination of the piece of messenger RNA added, the components would bind together on the ribosome
and be retained on the filter. If the sRNA failed to recognize the three-letter
message, everything would fall through the filter. Then when radioactivity was counted on the filter, none would be found. If that occurred, the
experiment would be repeated over and over again with different three-letter combinations until they found the right match. This greatly simplified

searching for which three-letter combination coded for which particular amino acid. What a contrast to the first UUUUUUUUUUUUUU experiment! Now Marshall needed to make all 64 three-letter combinations and test them. This foray into chemistry left Marshall well out of his comfort zone.

Of all the research associates to work on these problems, Joel Trupin and Don Kellogg had two of the most unusual starts to life. Trupin opined, "I spent my first six years on a collective farm, a Jewish anarchist collective farm, that started out in Michigan, lasted there for about four years, and then a fragment of the original group relocated to Virginia, where it lasted for another couple of years. So my first six years were on that collective farm."[57]

Kellogg's father, a noted biologist, as an experiment brought a monkey into the home when his son Don was a baby. He wanted to see if as his son learned to speak, the monkey would also acquire human language. The experiment failed. The monkey never learned to use human language. Don himself learned to speak but only at a later age than most other children[57]

Challenges dogged the intrepid researchers in Marshall's lab from every angle. Did each three-letter combination require a certain chemical modification on one end or the other to work properly?[58]This potentially added to their chemical quagmire of having to both make each three-letter combination and then add a minor change. If a particular three-letter combination resisted their efforts to make it, they had to find another way. And even then, they might still fail to make it.[59]

Finally, two bright spots emerged. One, the Gallard-Schlesinger Chemical Mfg. Corp. in New York, helped advance the research by offering chemicals for sale consisting of two-letter combinations to which a third letter could be added, greatly reducing the work involved. Marshall brought the whole batch.[60] The other involved Heppel at NIH and his postdoctoral student, Maxine Singer, who both jumped in to provide relief with their technical expertise.

Yet even now, Marshall fretted over getting the three-letter combination test right. Could better controls be used? Could ribosomes be better washed free of contaminants? What size ribosomes might work best? When an sRNA recognized a three-letter combination in the messenger RNA, could adjustments be made so that more ribosomes and radioactivity would be found on the filters? Could the three-letter combination *interfere* with the binding of sRNA?[61] Difficulties with any one of these questions could hamper comparisons from one experiment to the next.[62] Countless experiments would be needed to work out answers to each such question.

Growing increasingly testy, Marshall remonstrated himself: "Pick only 1 ... [problem] ... to concentrate on!!!! Give others away and follow partially."[63] Marshall planned to spend about 20 percent of his time reading and another 20 percent of his time just thinking about problems and their solutions. If the experiments worked well, he would not personally work on them. If they failed, he would work on them himself. However, he would not entrust reviewing everyone's data to anyone but himself.[64]

Marshall agonized over every aspect of the project. Even the source of water troubled him. He worried that minerals in glass containers might leak into the water used in his experiments. The minerals might then affect the results.[65] Despite progress being made, Marshall still thought inducing protein production was the best way to decipher the code.[66]

Marshall's meticulousness extended through the whole scientific process, from the generation of new ideas to final publication. "Where most of the world worried about the number of papers you published, Marshall didn't care about that. He cared about the quality of the paper. That was ingrained in you."[67]

Marshall oscillated back and forth over the correct combination of letters needed in the messenger RNA for proper sRNA recognition. Was it two-letters, three-letters, or a combination of both? In April 1964, Marshall, the experimentalist, still had his doubts. Six months later, he could not even say with certainty whether all combinations of three letters were read in their entirety or only partially.[68] Still unclear was another possibility. A three-letter combination might react with sRNA differently depending on whether the three-letter combination was in the middle of the messenger RNA or near one of the ends. Still unclear was the possibility of sRNA exchanges on the ribosomes, control of protein production, and how newly made protein got released from the ribosomes. All remained unknown.[69]

Crick faced no such crisis of conscience. For him, the operational details of the letter combinations were clear. As the experimental evidence grew, Crick modified his theories. Crick now found it obvious that similar three-letter combinations could code for one amino acid, that the message was read in groups of three letters from a fixed starting point, that the letter combinations in the message sequence were linear and parallel to the protein chain being made, that the same three-letter combinations were used by all organisms, that most of all coding combinations consisted of three letters, and that adjacent sets of three letters in the message did not overlap.[70] Crick thought if the laboratory experimentalists got moving, the code mess would straighten out. In 1963, when Crick wrote this, most of his details still lacked unambiguous evidence to support them.

By the time of the International Union of Biochemistry Congress in New York in 1964, Marshall's group had figured out how the three-letter code worked. The group had kept a blanket of secrecy over their work, so Marshall's presentation—filled with so much new information—thrilled the attendees. Even Crick might have been caught unawares, no easy task given his status as a scientific icon. Clark, one of Marshall's researchers, expressed sympathy about the shocked looks on the faces of Khorana's group from Wisconsin after the lecture.[32]

Even so, not everyone agreed with the use of a three-letter messenger. In Marshall's lab, O'Neal recalls that many of the experimental results were barely greater than those with the controls. This called into question how reliable the differences between the experiments and the controls might be. Initially, the work was subject to this criticism until confirmed by other labs.[28] Crick warned that attachment to ribosomes was not the same as making protein. He thought that Khorana's chemical approach was "probably the best evidence" to date and could be used to confirm Marshall's results.[71]

However, Crick's opinion did not stop him from pursuing Marshall and asking to see as-yet unpublished data. By now, Marshall had assembled most of the details of the genetic code. Marshall had earlier recognized how the third letter of each combination could vary. But it was Crick who garnered the priority of publication.

Crick called Pestka, who was still working with Marshall, rather than Marshall himself. Marshall had a sample of the first sRNA whose exact arrangement of all the letters in its structure had been deciphered by Robert Holley. Crick wanted Pestka to spill the details of how this sRNA worked in Marshall's experiments. Pestka, young but not foolish, asked Crick to call Marshall directly. Crick did call Marshall and got him to divulge his unpublished data. Marshall—naive, trusting, and intimidated—gave Crick what he wanted. Crick then turned around and published details about the variability of the third letter in each combination on his own.[72]

Crick's behavior differed from that found in conventional science in which data is shared only when parties agree to collaborate. Crick and Marshall had no collaborative agreement either orally or in writing. Crick considered his inquiries a collaboration.[73] Marshall did not. Crick's much more forceful personality helped magnify his accomplishments. The danger for Marshall lay in the fact that publication priority rules science. Consequently, Marshall, who was not boastful, also was no longer first to publish on the variability of the third letter. Marshall remained vulnerable to Crick. Marshall's career could be made or broken on the single printed date of a publication such as the variability of the third letter in the code.

When Crick sent a letter to Marshall and Khorana, he stated, "As you know, I have found myself involved in this [code work], but as a collator of information rather than a producer."[74]In this, Crick was correct. What Crick failed to mention, but Marshall certainly knew, was that Crick was a *self-appointed* collator who having obtained pre-publication material found no problem in "having to provide copies of my private version of the code to interested people." Crick justified his actions: "It is obvious that no one person has enough data to establish the code by himself, and also that by pooling all the information we can already arrive at most of the code."[75] Marshall, working night and day to establish the entire code, responded, "Why don't you write it yourself?"[75]

In spite of Crick's repeated interventions, Marshall could now see finishing the code work, and he felt impelled to work even harder. Everyone else in the lab became feverish with activity. Recalls O'Neal, "people came and went during the day, but I think you could honestly say the lab was going 18 hours a day. I was back many times at night, so was most of the group. ... And so I think we were all impressed with the importance of the work and ... [were] ... busy as beavers. ... I think the one reason that things worked out well is everybody was very ambitious, everybody was hardworking."[28]

In contrast, between 1962 and 1966, Crick delivered some 50 lectures on the genetic code at 30 different locations as far away as Vancouver, Canada, and Hyderbad, India. Arriving in the United States in early 1965, Crick telephoned Nirenberg to get his latest allocations of the code words. "It was a most exciting occasion for me," extolled Crick, "traveling about the country and seeing how various lines of evidence fitted together."[73]

Marshall, almost overwhelmed by work in the lab, had little time for such mad pursuits. Applications of the genetic code began to emerge. Marshall became interested, for example, in how an antibiotic interrupted protein synthesis. If an antibiotic interfered, bacteria could no longer make the proteins they needed and would die. Marshall explored whether the antibiotic interrupted the binding of the messenger to the ribosome.[76]

Zabriski Heaton, Marshall's lab technician, remained constantly busy. "Tabulating a summary of our results," she said, "as each ... [three-letter combination] ... was deciphered was challenging." Data poured in as each three-letter combination of messenger RNA was tested with each sRNA and the particular amino acid it carried. There were 64 possible three-letter combinations and each required several experiments to confirm for which sRNA and amino acid it coded. The data had to be arranged and organized. Zabriskie Heaton remembers, "I taped enough data paper together to create very large charts and drew the columns and rows with a ruler. Then, I painstakingly entered all the data from our experiments by hand. The resulting charts would become the 'Rosetta Stone of the Genetic Code' and some of them are now in the Smithsonian and the Library of Medicine."[17] Yet, it is often Crick who gets credit for making a chart of the genetic code.

Judith Levin, a member of Marshall's lab, remembers that "it was an incredible environment to be in. And I think that ... the focus of everyone's work and goal while we were there was to ... address very important questions. That was the hallmark of working with Marshall. ... Not to follow only the accepted dogma, but to explore things that seemed to be interesting and valid, even if they didn't quite go with the accepted ideas. ... Marshall was a very kind person," Levin went on to say. "He was a very gentle person. ... He was very driven, you know, in terms of his head."[3]

Marshall remained somewhat bemused by all the attention. "America," he recalled, "has been saying that my work may result in the cure for cancer and allied diseases, the cure for cancer and the end of mankind, and a better knowledge of the molecular structure of God." "Well," Marshall concluded, "it's all in a day's work."[77]

Hedging his bets, Marshall had early on noted, "the genetic code may *not* be universal; it may differ from species to species."[78] Marshall would later prove his own prophetic words incorrect. A research associate, Tom Caskey, would help him do it.

Caskey came to NIH in 1964. He had an opportunity to join one of several groups but ended up choosing Marshall. Caskey felt apprehensive about the competition from Khorana at the University of Wisconsin. Recalls Caskey, "We were in a horse race with him because the technology that we had developed was really simple ... and he had the capacity to do the chemical synthesis with the ... [three-letter combinations]. We were a bunch of biologists, molecular biologists. We were doing it by ... [using special proteins] ... and a wide variety of other methods. But he was a straightforward chemistry guy with a huge chemistry lab. So we had our work cut out for us."[79]

It would take Caskey and others several years after Marshall's pronouncement to show that the genetic code was the same in greatly diverse organisms.[80] Caskey also led a group within Marshall's lab to clarify how protein synthesis came to a natural stop at the end of the messenger RNA. [81] They expected to find a special sRNA that would recognize one of several three-letter combinations now known to mark the end of each protein chain. At that point, the production of the protein would stop. But they were in for a surprise. Stoppage occurred when special proteins, not an sRNA, recognized the three-letter combinations that brought protein production to a halt. "So that was really exciting. No one anticipated that we would find a protein that did that."[79]

Arthur Beaudet got his position in Marshall's lab by just calling up. His job was to capture sRNA from the livers of guinea pigs. To do this, Beaudet used a long glass tube packed with special material. The tube was so long that it extended through a hole from one floor in Marshall's lab to the floor below. Fluid with extracts of the liver cells entered the tube at the top. Some material stuck to the packing in the tube and some went through unattached. As fluid exited at the bottom of the tube, it was collected bit by bit and tested for the presence of sRNA.[82]

Edward Scolnick, another research associate, also participated in the successful search for the factors that stopped protein production:

I remember the first time Marshall popped in and said, "Come on in and tell me what you're doing." And I started to say to him, "Well, here's my data." And he said, "I don't want to see your data. Tell me how you did the experiment." I'll never forget this. "How did you do the experiment?" And I started to explain to him what I did, which wasn't what he wanted, still. He said, "No no, tell me from the beginning, how you did the experiment." In that meeting, he taught me how you really do science. The experimental approach. The bookkeeping. The solution books, the meticulousness with which you have to know what your … [chemicals] …, how you add them, the order in which you add them, the lack of cross-contamination of your … [chemicals]. I learned more in that hour with Marshall, than I had in all of my prior time in working in laboratories. It was an eye-opener.

That experience, that was it. I knew that I'd never be able to go back to medicine without doing research. It was such a high. … that you just say, "I want to do this over and over again in my life." There's nothing like this. We're discovering something fundamental about life and how cells work, and now I really do know how to do research in a rigorous way. It was just a life-changing experience. … I would never be in research if it weren't for Marshall Nirenberg."[67]

Scolnick went on to become president of Merck Research Laboratories.

Joseph Goldstein came to Marshall from Kingtree, South Carolina, a small town with a population of around 5,000 people. He may have been a small-town boy but he made a big impression on people. Robert Gallo, another NIH researcher, recalled, "I think Joe knew the data in papers I published better than I did. What a memory, and what a stickler for details, and … [an] enormous reader, [a] voracious [reader].[19] Goldstein joined Marshall who exposed him to the essence of scientific research. Goldstein must have been a quick study because he, in turn, shared a Nobel Prize with Michael Brown in 1985 for discoveries that led to the statin drugs for treating high cholesterol.

Goldstein said the transition at NIH from medicine to research took some doing. "In the very beginning, for the first few months, I was sort of lost, and then I found my way and … [my associates] … were really helpful. … It was intense and it was a lot of fun."[83] Goldstein has since remarked that nine Nobel laureates like him came out of the research program at NIH between 1964 and 1972.[84] Alfred Gilman was the other Nobel laureate to emerge from Marshall's lab. Goldstein says, "I do think that Marshall is sort of an unsung hero in the eyes of scientists. … I think it's … [because] … he didn't toot his own horn."[83]

Zabriskie Heaton recalled, "Manuscripts were written and rewritten, typed and retyped … often up until the last moment before the deadline. This was before the days of email and fax machines, so when Marshall and the secretary finished his paper for the Lasker Foundation award at 3 a.m. the morning of its deadline, Marshall left me a plane ticket, and I flew to New York and hand-delivered his paper to the Lasker Foundation head-quarters. The very next morning was Wednesday, October 16th, 1968, and it was announced that Marshall back at NIH had won the Nobel Prize."[17]

The mood at the lab that morning was buoyant and relieved. Marshall had won the prize everyone around him hoped he would. He had been awakened in the early morning hours with a call from Sweden announcing he would share the Nobel Prize with Robert Holley and Gobind Khorana. That morning in the lab, small sips of champagne were taken from lab glassware suddenly converted for that purpose. A sign hung in the hallway that trumpeted "UUU Are Great!" Marshall treated the entire staff to lunch in nearby Bethesda that afternoon.

A little later that month, Marshall and Perola met at the White House with President Lyndon Baines Johnson. Johnson had just come from Cabinet Room where he had convened a meeting with his advisors on the Vietnam War. Marshall had greatly benefited from the fallout of that war, which had sent research associates into his lab in lieu of going to Vietnam. Johnson must have been distressed from his meeting on the war's progress. Reaching into a drawer of his desk, he gave Marshall a box with a medal to commemorate his discovery of the genetic code.

After Marshall returned home, he found that Johnson had mistakenly given him instead a medal commemorating the Chamizal Settlement that ended a 100-year-long border dispute between Mexico and the United States. Disputed ownership of the Chamizal tract had remained a thorny issue between the two countries. Johnson's White House log makes no mention of either the giving or the returning of the medal.

In the end, Marshall took comfort from all he accomplished. "He knew," said Zabriskie Heaton, "that knowledge was what would last and endure for all eternity and that the knowledge we amassed was a legacy that would live on."[17]

Marshall initially resented, lamented, and then relented on attending the Nobel Prize ceremony in 1968. He considered a celebration of the Nobel Prize to be anticlimactic. The real game-changer had occurred years earlier. Then the instrument that counted radioactivity had spewed out large numbers upon the addition to his cell-free system first of the unnatural messenger RNA UUUUUUUUUUUUUU and then later just the three-letter combination UUU. With those two experiments, Marshall had finally unlocked the basics of how the genetic code worked.

He had immediately begun looking forward to exploring the biology of the nervous system, called neurobiology. He would spend the next 40 years in this new field. It was the frontier—the Wild West—of biological research. But that was not yet to be. Instead, Marshall would first have a week of travel and celebration as a mere diversion from his lab. Along with his wife, Perola, Marshall's sister Joan and his uncle Arthur traveled with him to Sweden.

In Stockholm on December 10th, Marshall attended a rehearsal in the Stockholm Concert Hall followed later by the prize presentation there, in the Grand Auditorium. The recipients were then presented to His Majesty King Gustav VI Adolf and members of the Swedish royal family, after which everyone sat down to a banquet in the Golden Hall at the City Hall. The following day, Marshall went to the office of the Nobel Foundation to pick up a check for $23,333, his share of the prize money. The remainder went to Ghobind Khorana and Robert Holley who shared the Prize for Physiology or Medicine with Marshall. The celebrations continued that evening with dinner at the Royal Palace hosted by the king. As on the previous day, Marshall had to put on full evening clothes.

On the third day of the festivities, in the auditorium of the Karolinska Hospital, Marshall, at 10:05 that morning, summarized in 35 minutes his blood, sweat, and tears of triumph over the past decade. Unlike his earlier experience at MIT, no one came forward this time after his talk to present their own slides on the code.

Neurobiology Comes to the Fore

Even then, Marshall's mind remained preoccupied with how the brain worked. He had already been thinking about the subject for almost a decade. Around October 1, 1959, entries on neurobiology first appear in Marshall's notebooks. At the time, only the barest outline of how cells produced protein had emerged. Discovery of messenger RNA lay in the future. Resolution of how letter combinations in messenger RNA led to the correct order of amino acids in proteins remained a fantasy.

Despite the lack of knowledge, Marshall laid down a plan to explore how the brain learned. He would inject into the brains of monkeys unnatural amino acids, which presumably would block production of protein. He might then train monkeys with and without such injections to learn a task. The brains of un-injected monkeys would continue to make proteins whereas the brains of the injected monkeys would not. What effect would blockage of protein production have on learning, Marshall wondered?[1]

Marshall had visualized working on brain-related projects ever since. Four years later, in the midst of contesting for control of the genetic code, his mind still wrapped around how the brain functioned. Again, he focused on memory. Gone was the use of monkeys. Perhaps his ongoing research with cell extracts and messenger RNA led him to simplify the problem of how the brain learns. He would use special proteins to carve out cells from the brain and instead grow the cells in the lab. There, he anticipated they would cluster together into thin sheets or balls to reform brain tissue. Marshall wanted to see how excitability in nerve cells affected RNA and protein production.[2]

What biochemical changes, he wondered, enabled the brain's nerve cells to connect to one another? Would the brains of older animals have more connections than younger ones? Most significantly, Marshall wondered, what constituted memory? Could memory be nothing more than the laying down of nerve pathways, each nerve containing one tiny bit of information?[2]

Marshall could not rein in his interest in the brain. Again and again, he toyed with the role of protein production in establishing memory.[3] He filled pages of his notebook with possible experiments. Then he countered with "criticisms" of why those ideas might not work. On other pages he wondered just how the brain develops? He imagined using animal brains at various stages of development and testing how their nerve pathways responded to electrical impulses. Basically, Marshall wanted to know when various activities of the brain become functional during development.[4] Perhaps, Marshall speculated, these electrical changes might represent an early form of memory.

How the genetic code might explain the inner workings of the brain constantly provoked Nirenberg's interest in neurobiology. The distribution of RNAs caught his interest.[5] Nerve cells are naturally stretched long. How much RNA clustered around the DNA in the nucleus of the nerve cell compared to the amount of RNA distributed outside the nucleus throughout the length of the cell? How much RNA might be found in one type of brain cell versus another type of brain cell? If he found differences, could the differences relate to the special functions of each cell? How much RNA could he find in the brain of a goldfish, as an experimental model, compared with RNA in just the retina of the goldfish eye? And he would not just use goldfish for his experiments. The nervous system of the cockroach, worm, mollusk, and cat, currently being explored and reported on by others, equally fascinated him.[6]

In 1963, in the midst of his work with unnatural messenger RNA and the genetic code, Marshall interviewed Norma Zabriskie Heaton to work with him as his technician. It was not the genetic code that he talked about with her. It was the use of the legs of cockroaches to study the nervous system. She did not like bugs, but she did like Marshall and so took the job. She stayed with him for 40 years. In the end, she never worked on a single cockroach leg.[7]

Once Marshall got the Nobel festivities out of the way, he settled down to explore the brain. Just as working on a home repair job requires the right tools, Marshall now knew that he also required the right tools to answer important questions about the brain. Those tools would be particularly important for the coming work in neurobiology. One critical tool would allow him to take the extraordinarily complex networks of a brain and reduce them to one simple network in the lab.

He teamed up with Phillip Nelson, who was also at NIH. Nelson was part of the Behavioral Biology Branch in the National Institute of Child Health and Human Development. Nelson held both an MD degree and a PhD degree in neuroscience from the University of Chicago. Marshall and Nelson, despite being at NIH at the same time, had not met. After all, NIH sits on more than 300 acres in Bethesda, Maryland. Rather, it took a meeting out in Boulder, Colorado, and an introduction by Eric Kandel to bring them together. Kandel would win the Nobel Prize in 2000 for how memory is stored in nerve cells.

Nelson grew cells taken directly from nervous tissue. The cells would grow for a while in the lab and then stop. When they discontinued growing, Nelson would have to re-prepare the cells all over again. This took time. It also caused confusion if two preparations of cells gave conflicting results in the same experiment. Working with the nervous system could be a frustrating business.

Where he once used bacterial cells, Marshall had confronted the fear that cell extracts would not replicate the production of protein found in intact cells. But he conquered that fear. Now there was a new one. Marshall fretted that nerve cells grown in the lab would lose their special functions. His concern rested on a long-held view of the brain. Scientists believed that once development of the brain ceased, the nerve pathways remained inviolate. That is, of course, until aging caused the brain to lose cells. Thus, Marshall and Nelson felt trepidation. If they freed nerve cells from their networks in the brain, might the cells cease their special functions?

The two men faced other technical concerns, as well. Extracting cells from brain gave two types of cells. The desired nerve cell or neuron was one. A support cell, the sort of "glue" that holds the nervous system together, was the other. Scientists wanted one, got both, and could not get rid of the other. Then Marshall and Nelson got wind of how just nerve cells could be obtained. At a meeting in Massachusetts, two other researchers shared about experiments they were running. They had eliminated the glue cell problem by extracting cells from a tumor of nerve cells in mice.

Tumor cells love to grow whether in the lab or in the body. Unlike healthy cells that only grow so long in the lab before dying off, tumor cells can live forever. This gives scientists a virtually unlimited supply of the same cells day after day, year after year. From the researchers they met in Massachusetts, Marshall and Nelson also got some hopeful news. The nerve cells from the tumors kept some expected biochemical characteristics even after growth in the lab.[8]

But did these cells show excitability of true nerve cells? Excitability is a hallmark of mature nerve cell function. Scientists already knew that "tickling" nerves cells with electricity causes them to become excited. This can be detected as a "hiccup" increase in voltage that nerve cells use to communicate with one another. Scientists call this phenomenon excitability.

In less than six months, Marshall and Nelson confirmed and extended the initial findings of the other lab. Remarkably, they discovered that these tumor nerve cells grown in the lab still exhibited excitability. Thus, the nerve cells might be functioning as they did in the body.[9] In less than two years, Marshall had already transitioned from one complex field of biology to a completely different and even more complex one.

By the start of 1971, Marshall and Nelson had found that a part of the genetic program that makes nerve cells excitable could also be transferred to cells not previously excitable.[10] The two types of cells merged together to become a single combined cell. The complexity of the nervous system had been reduced to a simple group of cells. Marshall was off and running. He could now apply what he had learned about bacteria and the genetic code to nerve cells that enabled brains to function.

Characterizing the electrical excitability and genetic transfer of excitability of nerve cells posed one small step for Marshall and Nelson. The next step became a giant leap. It took time, about five years to be exact. But they found something remarkable when they grew nerve and muscle cells together. The nerve cells reached out to the muscle cells and connected with them. In a little plastic dish 1.5 inches in diameter, Marshall and Nelson grew simple miniature nervous systems.[11] In the body, the connection of nerves and muscles enables movement of body parts, whether arms and legs, eyelids, or tongues.

As he had done with cell extracts from bacteria, Marshall now had a much simpler way of studying a complex biological phenomenon—the nervous system. Nelson recalls, Marshall "had a tremendously open mind, an acceptance to consider everything in all aspects of a situation. But at the same time, a tremendous rigor ... against ... accepting established things that weren't quite established. ... And he was just constantly probing for new ideas on how to do things."[12]

Marshall had once wondered about the amount of RNA in the retina of the goldfish eye. Now he could explore how nerve cells in the retina of the eye of chick embryos and adults organized themselves. He examined cells isolated from different places in the retina. He found that the amount of a particular protein produced in each isolated cell depended on where that cell had been located in the retina. The cell did not have to remain in the retina to show this behavior.[13]

To better understand the underpinnings of life, Marshall turned his attention to homeoproteins. About a decade earlier, these proteins had been discovered to affect development. Homeoproteins regulate the usage of information from DNA and do so by attaching to DNA at certain critical locations. Marshall found that the messenger RNA for one such protein became most abundant in 12-day-old mouse embryos and progressively decreased as development proceeded. The messenger RNA appeared in the brain but could also be found in tissues ranging from intestine to vertebrae.[14] Marshall went on to identify four new homeoproteins in mice and showed that during development, the amount of messenger RNA for each homeoprotein differs from one tissue to another.[15]

Marshall wanted to learn more about how the use of information in DNA affects development of embryos and their nerve pathways. He had used mice but decided he needed a simpler model organism. The mice required cages housed in rooms devoted just to animals. The mice also required constant maintenance: provisions of food and water, tests for diseases that can affect other mice, and sanitation. In the experiments he was now considering, the mouse embryos would also require larger amounts of valuable and costly RNAs that he planned to purchase.

So Marshall selected a different organism with which to experiment: fruit flies. Unlike mice, fruit flies are so much smaller and more easily handled. An adult fruit fly is the size of two pinheads. The flies can be housed in small Mason jars that easily sit on a desk. They exist on simple food consisting of a mixture of water, instant potato flakes, powdered milk, sugar, and yeast. Hundreds fit in one small jar. The fruit flies are not only inexpensive to grow and house but breed quickly, unlike mice. They also have one other important advantage. Their DNA matches about 75 percent of human DNA that can give rise to disease. So while Marshall might work with flies, what he learned could prove important for human health. Marshall decided to use fruit flies as the model organism for a host of studies on the nervous system.

Interfering RNA, a method developed only a few years earlier, provided a simpler research tool. Marshall had years ago foreseen how one type of RNA could interfere with use of specific messenger RNA. Interfering RNA gave substance to his vision. If the letters of the interfering RNA matched up with the letters of the messenger RNA, the latter would be unable to function. The match-up of letters would not be identical but, rather, complementary. Where messenger RNA had an A, the inhibitory RNA would have a U, and vice versa. Where one had as G the other would have a C.

This arrangement enabled the inhibitory RNA to cling to the messenger RNA. Marshall could make the match simply by knowing the exact chain of letters in each messenger RNA. Then he could use in the lab an inhibitory RNA with the complementary letters. The messenger RNA encoded an order of amino acids for one particular protein. If the messenger RNA could not work, the protein could not get made. Blocking the use of messenger RNA effectively prevented the use of that portion of information in DNA from which the messenger RNA had been copied.

Of particular interest to Marshall was a biochemical pathway named Hedgehog. A pathway is a coordinated network of steps inside a cell that leads to a certain product or result. The Hedgehog pathway interested Marshall because its cascade of signals guides early embryonic development.

Then the pathway closes down. If reactivated later in life, it can cause cancer. Past efforts to understand the role of DNA in this pathway gave unclear results. Marshall decided that RNA interference provided the tool to better investigate the effects caused by silencing portions of DNA.

He would use interfering RNA to block messenger RNA that contributed protein for the Hedgehog pathway. Marshall's first application of inhibitory RNA to development appeared as a collaboration in 2003. In the lab, the researchers grew cells derived from the larvae of fruit flies. The cells they chose could in larvae eventually give rise to the wings of the fly.[16] These studies provided more details about how the Hedgehog pathway controlled development.

In addition to cells of the fruit fly, Marshall also used the embryo. Obtaining the embryos entailed first isolating the freshly laid eggs of fruit flies. The embryos are roughly 6/1,000 of an inch. Microscopically thin glass tubes for injecting the embryos had to be prepared. Marshall used a device that simultaneously melted and pulled already thin tubes, stretching them further until they were reduced to the size of a human hair. Then a grinder was used to open the tips before the RNA was added. The tube was then used to inject the interfering RNA into the embryo. All of this work with fruit flies was exacting. It had to be done with a microscope, good eyesight, and a very steady hand. The inhibitory RNA affected those portions of DNA that are directly or indirectly involved in the development of the nervous system.[17]

Personal Loss and Recovery

Ironically, as Marshall pursued how the brain develops and functions, his beloved wife Perola developed Alzheimer's disease. Now sadly familiar to many families, Alzheimer's is a type of dementia that causes problems with memory, thinking, and behavior. The causes are unclear, diagnosis is difficult, and treatment nearly impossible. The disease progresses slowly but irreversibly. Symptoms get worse with time. Marshall cared for Perola over her extended illness of ten years. Extraordinarily loyal, Marshall changed his whole life during that period to tend to her. He did not travel but just worked every day at NIH and came home to Perola at night. She died in 2001.

Perola's death left Marshall grief stricken, and he no longer found pleasure in his scientific forays. That year, however, he did manage to sign a letter to President George W. Bush along with 79 other Nobel Laureates. The letter may have carried the largest collection of Nobel Laureate signatures ever sent to a president. The Laureates sought to soften Bush's opposition to the use of federal funds for stem cell research. At the time, scientists derived stem cells from human embryos discarded at fertility clinics. Stem cells, then as now, may potentially help cure brain disorders and diseases, as well as lead to replacement of tissues and organs.[18]

Shortly after Perola's death, Marshall struggled to get his life back in order. Uncharacteristically, for he preferred time in the lab, he traveled to Philadelphia to attend a meeting. There, he met a friend who shared with him the unexpected death of her spouse years earlier. She had remarried and urged Marshall to consider doing the same. She had a friend, Myrna Weissman, whose husband had also died unexpectedly. She asked Marshall to call Weissman.

Weissman held a distinguished academic post in New York City. She has emphasized that the Civil Rights Movement of the 1960s brought about legislation that opened doors for woman in terms of educational opportunities and careers. As a young mother with four small children, she had been admitted, albeit somewhat reluctantly, into a PhD program at Yale to study epidemiology—how chronic disease spreads and can be controlled. Weissman went on to compile an impressive list of accomplishments. She has authored 550 scientific articles and chapters, written 11 books, and won about 14 awards in the process. A member of the Institute of Medicine, she focuses on mood and anxiety disorders using a host of methods to understand, treat, and prevent these disorders.[19]

Years earlier, Weissman, married with three children, had worked at NIH as did her husband at the time. She had heard about Marshall but had never met him. But she did meet Perola. Weissman, pregnant with her fourth child, caught the attention of Perola in the cafeteria one day. At the time, few pregnant women worked at NIH. Weissman recalled that Perola "came up to me and made some very friendly comment. ... I knew her name and realized she was married to Marshall Nirenberg. ... I knew he was a legend there. I realized it, but I never saw her again. She was a lovely woman. A very beautiful woman. Very graceful, lovely."[19]

After returning from Philadelphia, Marshall called Weissman in late December. But it took four months before they finally got together in New York City. Because her second husband had died, Weissman hesitated to date Marshall who was nine years her senior. Their first date included a long walk and talk through Central Park and dinner. Eventually their budding friendship blossomed into love and the two were married in 2005. The marriage greatly altered Marshall's life in the following years. Childless before, he now had four stepchildren and grandchildren as well. Marshall loved children and reveled in this newfound life experience.

Continuing on with Research

Using many different examples of interfering RNA, Marshall and his group had previously found 43 cases of inhibitory RNA blocking development of the embryonic nervous system in fruit flies. Now they added 22 more. The total here and in the previous study means they had tested about half of the total DNA in fruit flies responsible for protein production.[20]

As publications poured forth from his lab, Marshall requested an increase in salary. In 2006, his proposed salary reached $180,000, an increase of $33,015 over what he had been earning. Marshall's father, Harry Nirenberg, would have been proud to know that his son had been able to earn a substantial living as a biochemist. His mother, Minerva, knew nothing of Marshall's success, having died of cancer in 1960. Harry had finally achieved financial success after converting his farm to commercial warehouses, but the loss of Minerva was difficult for Harry to bear, and he took his own life in 1961. He had, however, lived to see Marshall's triumph in Moscow.

The loss of his wife Perola to Alzheimer's disease motivated Marshall even more to understand the biological basis of memory. He studied another pathway, a coordinated network of steps inside cells. This pathway posed a potential target for therapies designed to enhance human memory. Marshall's research group screened about 73,000 compounds and identified 1,800 with the desired drug activity. These drugs enhanced a sequence of signals in the cell thought to be important for long-term memory.[21]

Marshall was the first to use the nerve cells he had developed for growth in the lab to spell out how drugs used for pain also can become addictive. He had started these studies in 1974. Over the course of three decades and several papers, Marshall pushed the boundaries of the biology of addiction. Marshall showed that drugs like morphine affect a key protein in the cell. As a result, making nerve cells addicted to morphine required the production of this protein in the cells. Marshall had dreamed of experiments on protein production in nerve cells decades earlier. Now these experiments had turned his dreams into reality. Testing more than a thousand compounds, his group discovered eight potent agents that could block addiction.[22]

Just as Marshall used his lab to conduct experiments and advance knowledge in neurobiology, Crick used his offices to meet with neurobiologists and learn from them. Appointed in 1976 to the staff of the Salk Institute in La Jolla, California, Crick had the time and resources to pursue that strategy.[23] Now he prepared to plunge into the biology of the brain. Three years later, he was still gathering information from experts in the field. Not surprisingly, Crick found this new field challenging.

Eventually, Crick switched into neurobiology as Marshall had done earlier. In the late 1970s, the editors of *Scientific American* planned a special
issue on the brain. As they had done before with the genetic code, the editors passed on covering the notable achievements in brain biology already
made by Marshall over the past decade. Marshall was still a newcomer to
the field and would remain in neurobiology research for the next 30 years.

Instead, they called on Crick who had barely gotten into the field. In his
article, Crick claimed to have been interested in the biology of the brain for
more than 30 years, but only in the last two years "attempted to study it
seriously."[24] However, there is little record to support Crick's prior interest.
At the time of the article, in fact, Crick had not published a single significant paper in neurobiology.

Perhaps *Scientific American* hoped that Crick would furnish a much more
provocative article than Marshall would. After all, several years earlier, with
Leslie Orgel, another member of the RNA Tie Club, Crick published a paper
that described the "theory that organisms were deliberately transmitted to
Earth by intelligent beings on another planet."[25] Crick supposedly did not
believe the idea. Years later, he admitted he had not a shred of evidence to
support it.

Exactly why Crick entered neurobiology is unclear. It occurred around
the time that he emigrated from the United Kingdom due to a change in
the tax laws. The change would have made Crick unable to keep a significant portion of his overseas earnings from lectures and awards when
he returned home.[26] As a result, Crick ended up at the Salk Institute in
California. Two years into his appointment there, Crick apparently committed himself to neuroscience. Perhaps his associates convinced him that
neurobiology remained the last "frontier" of biology. Perhaps Marshall's
successful entry into neurobiology a decade earlier caught Crick's attention.

For both Marshall and Crick, change was *not* inevitable. Crick clung to
his theoretical approach to scientific problems. Marshall favored experimental methods. Crick no longer had Jim Watson or Sydney Brenner from
the RNA Tie Club at his side. Marshall no longer had Leon Heppel, Phil
Leder, or Tom Caskey with whom he had worked on the genetic code. The
scientific legacies that Marshall and Crick would leave to the neurosciences
would now depend largely on each man alone. Marshall had no use for
theory, whereas Crick had every use for experimental findings to support
his ideas.

In 1980, Crick began working on a theory of dreams. Three years later,
he published a paper on it with a coauthor. In it, they proposed that dream
sleep reversed the way learning took place in the brain. The dream process

eliminated unnecessary patterns of nerve cell interactions in the part of the brain responsible for memory, attention, perceptual awareness, thought, language, and consciousness.[27]

About four years later, Crick fastened onto the one subject that would occupy the rest of his life. He would focus on where consciousness is centered in the brain. His first step toward tackling the subject of consciousness came in a paper on how the brain works with the eye to focus attention.[28] Crick thought the process involved a region of the brain called the thalamus. Three years later, two authors confirmed Crick's basic idea.[29]

Eventually collaborating with Cristof Koch, a man 40 years younger, Crick focused on the basis for consciousness in the brain.[30] The two men later constructed a framework based on two assumptions: first, that consciousness required a scientific explanation and, second, that "all the different aspects of consciousness … employ a common mechanism or perhaps a few such mechanisms."[31] They portrayed consciousness as synchronized excitability of all the nerve cells anywhere in the brain involved in the perception of a particular event.[32] Enunciated in 1994, Crick abandoned the idea in 2003.

In the 25 years that he devoted to the brain and consciousness, Crick alone and with Koch published 23 papers and short articles on consciousness. The aim of many of them was to attract more researchers to the study of consciousness. Eventually, the two authors settled on a part of the brain called the claustrum as the site of consciousness.[33] To test their theory, all or part of the claustrum would have to be removed either transiently or permanently. Unfortunately, this could not be done. Surgery or drugs are ineffective for solely inactivating the claustrum. Thus, there are no experiments to support Crick's hypothesis. Today, however, consciousness still remains an area of interest in neuroscience.[34]

Over a 40-year period, Marshall studied the biology and function of the brain. He used organisms ranging from chickens and fruit flies to mice. His prodigious output of research averaged almost three papers a year over that time span. The impact of his findings is yet to be fully recognized. Today, for example, ongoing research is looking at reprogramming normal adult skin and liver cells, among others, to become various types of nerve cells. Homeoproteins, similar to the ones Marshall studied, figure prominently in changing cells from one type to another.[35] These studies may eventually lead to replacing nerve cells, spinal cords, or parts of the brain damaged by disease or other factors. Marshall could not help his wife Perola survive Alzheimer's disease. But he leaves a legacy in neurobiology that may one day help many, many others.

11 Reversions

Veteran's Day 2009 had passed gray and gloomy, but by evening, the stars had come out. It was an altogether fitting day for the event Marshall had planned.

The day had been highlighted by President Barack Obama's visit on the rainy 11th day of the 11th month to Arlington National Cemetery. There at the 11th hour in the morning, he laid a wreath at the Tomb of the Unknowns. Afterwards, President Obama visited section 60 where troops who had died fighting wars in Iraq and Afghanistan were interred.

By 6:30 that evening, the thin veneer of wet despair that hovered over the nation's capital all day began to lift. The somber mood of the day dissipated, and the light of a fading full moon took its place.

Well-dressed people streamed up the curved driveway to the light-filled front door of the Cosmos Club at 2121 Massachusetts Avenue Northwest. Notable among them was Marshall, a relatively tall former Floridian with a large shock of white hair. About seven months earlier, he had just passed his 82nd birthday. Marshall had planned a reception at the Cosmos Club that evening for friends, family, and colleagues.

In 1968, Marshall had been one of three to win the Nobel, the highest prize awarded for scientific achievement. Now he was in the twilight of his life. Fifty years earlier, Marshall had embarked on an intellectual voyage to ferret out how cells use inherited information from DNA. Marshall's success in completing that voyage, despite waves of uncertainty and foul winds of competitors, marked him as an immortal of science.

Marshall had planned this special occasion to relive one more time the momentous events that had unexpectedly shaped and filled his life—along with a select number of his guests. Many of the people arriving at the Cosmos Club that night, once young men and women in the prime of their lives, had worked to define the genetic code. They had shared Marshall's frustrations and joys, his failures and triumphs. Now, together again once more, they too, far removed from their youth, would soon be tottering on the cold cusp of old age.

In Washington, D.C., famous for the "Type A" personalities of its denizens, the Cosmos Club stands as a paean to high achievers. It was a perfect setting for this event. Among the members of the Cosmos Club, over the years, have been three U.S. presidents, two vice presidents, a dozen Supreme Court justices, 32 Nobel Prize winners, 56 Pulitzer Prize winners, and 45 recipients of the Presidential Medal of Freedom.[1] However, Marshall chose not to include his name among them.

The Cosmos Club occupies what was once known as the Townsend Mansion. The mansion is one of the jewels of Washington's Embassy Row. Standing on a site of almost one acre at 2121 Massachusetts Avenue and flanked by gardens, the mansion is one of the great turn-of-the-century residences that give Massachusetts Avenue its stateliness. The Dupont Circle area today is close by the heart of nightlife in the District.

Dupont Circle became Washington's most fashionable address in the last quarter of the 19th century. The development of what had been an outlying area of working class shanties, slaughterhouses, and a brickyard was spurred by the public works improvements inaugurated in the early 1870s.

Within the next several decades Dupont Circle became ringed with the mansions of families who had made their fortunes elsewhere but wished to establish a social presence in the nation's capital. One such family included Mary Scott Townsend, who exemplified this "upper crust" of society. Townsend as an heiress to a fortune, and enjoying great wealth, bought the property and substantial residence that the Cosmos Club eventually purchased from her daughter in 1950.[2] So vastly different was life in the Gilded Age when Mary Scott Townsend lived there that what then served as a home for a family of three today serves as a club for several thousand members.

Guests arriving for Marshall's reception clambered up the few original granite steps leading from the sidewalk to the driveway set with the original limestone parapet and marked with elaborately carved limestone vases. They encountered a building of elegant French Renaissance structure, inspired by the style of Louis XVI, standing amid ancient wisteria and magnolia trees. The three-and-a-half story central block of the building towered over them, flanked further on each side by a two-story wing, each crowned with balustrade parapets. They entered through a central door marked with a cast iron and glass roof.

Crossing the entrance hall with its notable marble construction, the guests went up the curved staircase with its rich red carpet and splendid wrought iron railing to the second floor. Marshall's reception encompassed two dining rooms and an adjoining alcove.

While others planned the reception, they needed Marshall's acceptance to hold the reception at the Cosmos Club. Had the reception been held 25 years earlier, Marshall would not have agreed. A sense of great modesty and a strong social conscience guided Marshall's actions. Despite the Cosmos Club's emphasis on members of exceptional accomplishment, Marshall had declined to join.

To those who knew him, the reasons were obvious. Even before he gained fame for winning the Nobel Prize, Marshall believed that scientists were accountable to society. Addressing the future of scientific inquiry in a handwritten note in 1966, Marshall invoked the words of eminent virologist Salvador Luria. He said, "The impact of science on human affairs imposes on its practitioners an inescapable responsibility."[3]

Anticipating the ethical and moral implications of genetic research in a 1967 editorial in *Science*, Marshall noted the expansion of scientific knowledge could soon lead to man's "power to shape his own biological destiny. Such power can be used wisely or unwisely, for the betterment or detriment of mankind." Marshall further stated, "When man becomes capable of instructing his own cells, he must refrain from doing so until he has sufficient wisdom to use this knowledge for the benefit of mankind."[3]

Over his career, Marshall had also used his scientific stature to protest the political repression and detention of scientists around the world. With a colleague, he protested the Brazilian government's purging of three of its renowned scientists. In a letter to the then president of Brazil, the two scientists argued for the continuity between the scientific exchange of ideas and political freedom. They noted that Brazil's actions would certainly result in "serious repercussions among scientists in the world community, whose sympathy and cooperation is essential to the continued technological development of Brazil."[3]

Marshall regularly lent his support and name to strengthen various environmental and humanitarian causes or to speak out on fundamental political issues. Marshall was one of 80 Nobel Laureates who issued the "Manifesto Against Hunger" in 1981, calling for the worldwide end of starvation. The following year, Marshall supported the "Declaration on Prevention of Nuclear War," presented to Pope John Paul II by an assembly of presidents of scientific academies and scientists from all over the world.[3]

Twenty-five year earlier, Marshall had reason not to join the Cosmos Club. From the date of its founding in 1878 and for the next 110 years, the Club had systematically excluded women from its membership. Back then, the Cosmos Club required that a woman enter through a rear door. She then would proceed a short distance to a sort of "holding" room where she would patiently wait as a guest. When the gentleman who had invited her appeared, he would escort her to the dining or meeting rooms.

At the end of December 1972, a drive to get women admitted to the Cosmos Club failed. One member who collected 60 signatures on a petition to get women admitted knew that that the petition would not succeed. And it did not.[4]

Eight years later, the 101-year-old men's society again overwhelmingly rejected a proposal to admit women as members. "Members who spearheaded the effort to admit qualified women [later said] the issue is probably dead for years to come. Though none would comment for the record, some club officials and members privately expressed delight at the result. 'If God had wanted women to be members,' wrote one member on his ballot, 'He would have made them men.'... If you don't like [the rules] get out, but leave the rest of us in peace."[5]

But the issue of admitting women refused to go quietly.[6] The final successful vote to admit women came only after years of continuing controversy. The D.C. Human Rights Office held that anyone who receives a business license from the District government must comply with the city's antidiscrimination law. The Office found "probable cause to believe" that the all-male Cosmos Club violated the law by barring women as members.[7] The Office urged the club in 30 days to change its 109-year-old policy.

Considering that African-Americans constituted about 70 percent of the population of the District of Columbia at the time, one might have expected the District of Columbia to have been especially sensitive to issues of discrimination long before 1987. Apparently, where women were involved, it was not.[7]

With these revolutionary changes at the Cosmos Club, plans for Marshall's reception there later became viable. Marshall asked his former partners in the genetic code research to join him and they did. Many flew in from around the country. Though a weekday event, the invitees unhesitatingly left their academic positions; executive suites; retirements, grandchildren, and daily routines to join Marshall for a never-to-be forgotten evening at the Cosmos Club.

Invitations went out to more than 350 people who had helped to define Marshall's life and career. They included 110 who had worked with Marshall in neurobiology, the field in which he spent the bulk of his career. At the time of the reception, Marshall also had 11 scientific staff in his lab. If one added in the 29 medical and postdoctoral graduates who had worked on the genetic code, Marshall had trained about 150 scientists over the course of his career. It was a stunningly large number and one in which he took great pride.

Despite that number, Marshall had resisted getting directly involved in education at an academic institution. He always wanted to focus on his research and not spend time in other academic activities including teaching and committee work. Yet regardless of which field he worked in, he always drew to his lab bright and ambitious young scientists in search of the best possible training and experience and eager to start their careers.

Invitations went out to a far-flung group of friends and family from all over the country. Myrna Weissman, Marshall's second wife, proffered invitations to her family, friends, and associates to join the festivities. Marshall also invited 36 colleagues with whom he had worked, collaborated, or befriended at NIH.

After time for social mixing—since many attendees had not seen Marshall or each other for many years—the evening program began. Marshall gave replicas of the Nobel Prize medals to 27 of his former lab colleagues from his genetic code days. Made of solid brass and weighing a little over half a pound, each measured about three inches in diameter. On one side, raised letters stated "National Institutes of Health, Molecular Biology Medal, 2009." Inscribed on the reverse side were the words, "For Contributions To Deciphering The Genetic Code Or The Mechanism Of Protein Synthesis" followed by the name of the recipient. Each replica was set in a small display case.

Those at the reception who had worked on the problems of the genetic code had helped Marshall race to find answers. They had come to work with him and knew that if successful, solving a problem of this magnitude might warrant a Nobel Prize. When the Nobel award came in 1968, it was a triumph for all concerned. What would have happened to all of them gathered there that night if Severo Ochoa—himself a Nobel Laureate—and his group at NYU had managed to outwit Marshall? What if the RNA Tie Club had scored a coup with one of their theories?

Afterwards, the guests proceeded to the members' dining area where a long table had been provisioned with fried oysters, crab morsels, wild mushroom tartlets, sliced roast tenderloin, herbed salmon, sliced ham, roasted turkey, Viennese and mini pastries, vegetable crudités, and assorted fruits and cheeses. A bar offered wine, mineral water, soft drinks, and assorted juices. Cocktail tables scattered about had been each set with a votive candle.

As the clock struck 9:30 that evening, the reception drew to a close. Marshall and his wife Myrna quietly departed for their home in Potomac, Maryland. Unknown to most at the festive gathering, Marshall and Myrna harbored a tragic secret. Marshall had always been a very private person and did not wish to disclose this news.

That night, his handsome shock of white hair was actually a wig to hide his embarrassment, because chemotherapy had robbed him of his own hair. Marshall had recently been a patient at the Memorial Sloan-Kettering Cancer Center in New York City. There, despite the best possible treatment medicine had to offer, Marshall had not received a favorable prognosis. The night of his reception, Marshall knew that he was terminally ill. On January 15, 2010, just a little more than two months after the festive Cosmos Club event, Marshall died at the age of 82 from a rare form of intestinal cancer.

That Marshall, friendly but quiet and modest, had become a scientist surprised no one who knew him: that he eventually won a Nobel Prize surprised almost everyone. Marshall appeared in life's early stages to be—in every sense of the word—a least likely man. Unlike many of his peers, he showed no early promise of such an achievement. He made no unusual academic ripples in high school. He did not enter college early or graduate with an armful of awards. He did not go to an outstanding graduate school or achieve unusually high marks and engender faculty admiration. Thus, Marshall's story is everyone's story and not just the story of a Nobel Laureate.

Notes

Introduction

1. Ridley, M., *Francis Crick: Discoverer of the Genetic Code*, Atlas Books, Harper/Collins, New York, 2006.

2. Sydney Brenner, DPhil, Howard Hughes Medical Institute, http://www.hhmi.org/scientists/sydney-brenner.

Chapter 1

1. *New York Times*, January 1, 1927, p. 1.

2. Ibid, p. 5.

3. Cornell University, Medical Center Archives, http://www.med.cornell.edu/archives/history/ny_nursery.html?name1=New+York+Nursery+and+Child's+Hospital&type1=2Active.

4. Charles Lindbergh Flies Solo across the Atlantic, The Learning Network, May 21, 1927, http://learning.blogs.nytimes.com/2012/05/21/may-21-1927-charles-lindbergh-flies-solo-across-the-atlantic/comment-page-1.

5. *New York Times*, January 2, 1928, p. 31.

6. *New York Times*, October 12, 1927, p. 20.

7. Brest Litovsk from the Jewish Encyclopedia, JewishGen Belaurus Sig., http://www.jewishgen.org/belarus/je_brest_litovsk.htm.

8. Homage to Odessa, Beit Hatfutsot, The Musuem of the Jewish People, http://www.bh.org.il/on-line-exhibition-intro.aspx?45474.

9. *New York Times,* September 22, 1929, p. 28.

10. The Stock Market Crash of 1929, About.Com 20th Century History, http://history1900s.about.com/od/1920s/a/stockcrash1929.htm.

11. Farming in the 1930s, Wessels Living History Farm, http://www.livinghistory farm.org/farminginthe30s/money_01.html.

12. Harris, R., Marshall Nirenberg Interview, National Library of Medicine, 1995–1996.

13. Nirenberg, J., Eulogy for Marshall Nirenberg, January 19, 2010.

14. Razeghi, A., *Hope: How Triumphant Leaders Create the Future*, Jossey-Bass, San Francisco, CA, 2006.

15. Fowler, J.K., On the Association of Affections of the Throat with Acute Rheumatism *The Lancet* 2:933–934, 1880.

16. Veasy, L.G., Rheumatic Fever and Streptococcal Infection: Unraveling the Mysteries of a Dread Disease, *New England Journal of Medicine* 338:926, 1998.

17. Reeves, C., Rheumatic Fever in America and Britain: A Biological, Epidemiological, and Medical History, *Medical History* 45:296–297, 2001.

18. Stollerman, G.H., Rheumatic Fever, *The Lancet* 349:935–942, 1997.

19. Garvey, M.A., Giedd, J., and Swedo, S.E., PANDAS: The Search for Environmental Triggers of Pediatric Neuropsychiatric Disorders: Lessons from Rheumatic Fever, *Journal of Child Neurology* 13:413–423, 1998.

20. Shader, M., interview with author, June 19, 2012.

Chapter 2

1. Total and Foreign-Born Population, New York City 1790–2000, http://www.nyc .gov/html/dcp/pdf/census/1790-2000_nyc_total_foreign_birth.pdf.

2. Streamliner Schedule, Official Guide December 1941, http://www.streamliner schedules.com/concourse/track2/orangeblossom194112.html.

3. Thomson, H.B., Orlando's Martin Andersen: Power Behind the Boom, *The Florida Historical Quarterly* 79:492–516, 2001.

4. Florida (State) Work Projects Administration, Federal Works Agency, *Florida: A Guide to the Southernmost State*, Oxford University Press, New York, 1939.

5. City of Orlando Economic Development, City Planning Division, www.cityof orlando.net//planning/cityplanning/default.html.

6. *Washington Post*, January 24, 1937, p. F5.

7. Camp, Paul D., A Study of Range Cattle Management in Alachua County, Florida, Bulletin 246, June 1932, University of Florida, Agricultural Experiment Station, Gainesville, Florida.

8. Orlando, Jewish Virtual Library, http://www.jewishvirtuallibrary.org/jsource/judaica/ejud_0002_0015_0_15198.html.

9. Honoree Is Living Link to Most of the 20th Century, *Orlando Sentinel*, http://articles.orlandosentinel.com/2002-09-29/news/0209270503_1_wittenstein-van-arsdel-florida-history.

10. Maury Road, Orlando, Florida, Google Maps, http://maps.google.com.

11. Boyles, J., interview with author, February 8, 2013.

12. Harris, R., Marshall Nirenberg Interview, National Library of Medicine, 1995–1996.

13. Bonnheim, B., personal communication.

14. New York City, Department of City Planning, New York City Land Use, http://www.nyc.gov/html/dcp/html/landusefacts/landusefactshome.shtml

15. Shofner, J.H., *Orlando: The City Beautiful*, Continental Heritage Press, Tulsa, Oklahoma, 1984, p. 27.

16. Ibid, pp. 28–29.

17. Ibid, p. 102.

18. Ibid, p. 104.

19. Ibid, p. 106.

20. Rise in Orlando's Population of 10,000 Since 1930 Seen, *Wall Street Journal*, December 12, 1938, p. 8.

21. Shofner, *Orlando: The City Beautiful*, p. 116.

22. Marshall Nirenberg papers, National Library of Medicine, Pittman, J. to Nirenberg M.W., March 9, 1996.

23. Freedom Never Dies: The Legacy of Harry T. Moore, Public Broadcasting Service, http://www.pbs.org/harrymoore/terror/k.html.

24. Archer, K., The Limits to the Imagineered City: Sociospatial Polarization in Orlando, *Economic Geography* 73:322–336, 1997.

25. Porter, T.M., Segregation and Desegregation in Parramore: Orlando's African American Community, *The Florida Historical Quarterly* 82:289–312, 2004.

26. Brotemarkle, B.D., Crossing Division Street: A History of the African American Community in Orlando, Florida, UMI Microform 3069747 Dissertation.

27. Shields, Dennis A., Consolidation and Concentration in the U.S. Dairy Industry, Congressional Research Service, Washington, D.C., 2010.

Chapter 3

1. Kinzie, J., Palmer, M., Hayek, J., Hossler, D., Jacob, S.A., and Cummings, H., *Fifty Years of College Choice: Social, Political, and Institutional Influences on the Decision-Making Process*, Lumina Foundation for Education, New Agenda Series, vol. 5, no. 3, September 2004, p. 6.

2. University of Florida Catalog, 1945–1946.

3. Blocker, A. and R., interview with author, November 14, 2012.

4. Becker, S., interview with author, June 14, 2012.

5. Deutsch, A., Lincoln's Legacy: Land-Grant Colleges and Universities, *Carnegie Reporter,* Winter 2012, http://carnegie.org/publications/carnegie-reporter/single/view/article/item/318.

6. Virgil Hawkins Story, Levin College of Law, University of Florida, http://www.law.ufl.edu/about/about-uf-law/history/virgil-hawkins-story.

7. Shaw, J.S., A Breathe of Fresh Air in College Rankings, The John William Pope Center for Higher Education Policy, May 18, 2008, http://www.popecenter.org/commentaries/article.html?id=2006.

8. Boyles, J., interview with author, February 8, 2013.

9. Hillman, A., interview with author, January 16, 2012.

10. Harris, R., Marshall Nirenberg Interview, National Library of Medicine, 1995–1996.

11. Platnick, N.I., Peter J. Solomon Family Curator of Spiders, Division of Invertebrate Zoology, American Museum of Natural History, personal communication, March 3, 2010.

12. Geiger, J., interview with author, December 13, 2010.

13. Bassett, M., archivist, Barnard College, March 17, 2010.

14. John Carter, registrar, Columbia University, April 1, 2010.

15. Nicole Milano, assistant, New York University Archives, April 7, 2010.

Chapter 4

1. Holton, R., Remembrance of Marshall Nirenberg, letter to Minor Judd Coon, April 16, 2011, http://www.biochem.med.umich.edu/files/Holton%20remembrances%20of%20Nirenberg.pdf.

2. Wagner, C., interview with author, April 5, 2011.

3. Coon, M.J., interview with author, May 6, 2011.

Chapter 5

1. Olby, R., *Francis Crick: Hunter of Life's Secrets*, Cold Spring Harbor Laboratory Press, Cold Spring Harbor, New York, 2009, p. 245.

2. Gallo, R., interview with author, May 26, 2011.

3. Watson, J., *The Double Helix*, Athenum, New York, 1968, p. 1.

4. Olby, *Francis Crick*, p. 255.

5. Watson, J.D. and Crick, F.H.C., Genetical Implications of the Structure of Deoxyribonucleic Acid, *Nature* 171:964–967, 1953.

6. Sanger, F. and Thompson, E.O., The Amino-acid Sequence in the Glycyl Chain of Insulin, *Biochemical Journal* 53:353–366, 1953.

7. Ridley, M., *Francis Crick: Discoverer of the Genetic Code*, Atlas Books, Harper/Collins, New York, 2006, p. 85.

8. Portugal, F.H. and Cohen, J.S., *A Century of DNA*, MIT Press, Cambridge, 1977, p. 291.

9. Harris, R., Marshall Nirenberg Interview, National Library of Medicine, 1995–1996.

10. Aspaturian, H., interview with Seymour Benzer, http://oralhistories.library .caltech.edu/27.

11. Felesenfeld, G., interview with author, November 20, 2012.

12. Olby, *Francis Crick*, pp. 188–190.

13. Watson, J.D. and Crick, F.H.C., Molecular Structure of Nucleic Acids, *Nature* 171:737–738, 1953.

14. Olby, *Francis Crick*, pp. 290–292.

15. Marshall Nirenberg Papers, National Library of Medicine, Box 22, D7, VIIA, September 1959–May 1960, September 24, 1959.

16. McElroy, W.D. and Glass, B., eds., *The Chemical Basis of* Heredity, Johns Hopkins Press, Baltimore, 1957, p. 748.

17. Marshall Nirenberg Papers, National Library of Medicine, Box 22, D7, VIIA, September 1959–May 1960, p. 21.

18. Lesson Page; Uncertainty: Possible Combinations, Oswego City School District, http://www.studyzone.org/testprep/math4/d/possiblecombinationl.cfm.

19. George Gamow to Linus Pauling, October 22, 1953, Ava Helen and Linus Pauling Papers, Oregon State University Libraries, http://scarc.library.oregonstate.edu/coll/pauling/dna/corr/sci9.001.43-gamow-lp-19531022-05.html.

20. Crick, F.H.C., On Degenerate Templates and the Adaptor Hypothesis, http://profiles.nlm.nih.gov/ps/access/SCBBGF.pdf.

21. Brenner, S., On the Impossibility of All Overlapping Triplet Codes in Information Transfer from Nucleic Acids to Proteins, *Proceedings of the National Academy of Sciences of the United States of America* 43:687–694, 1957.

22. Crick, F.H.C., The Present Position of the Coding Problem, *The Brookhaven Symposia in Biology* 12:35–39, 1958.

23. Gamow Symposium, Rich, A., Gamow and the Genetic Code, 115–122, the George Gamow Symposium, vol. 129, Eamon Harper and David Anderson, eds., American Scientific Publishers, Valencia, California, 1997.

24. Olby, *Francis Crick*, p. 232.

25. Linus Pauling to George Gamow, December 9, 1953, Ava Helen and Linus Pauling Papers, Oregon State University Libraries, http://scarc.library.oregonstate.edu/coll/pauling/dna/corr/sci9.001.43-gamow-lp-19531022-05.html.

.26. Marshall Nirenberg Papers, National Library of Medicine, Box 22, D6, VIA, 1958, November, p. 139.

27. Hoagland, M.B., Stephenson, M.L., Scott, J.F., Hecht, L.I. and Zamecnik, P.C., A Soluble Ribonucleic Acid Intermediate in Protein Synthesis, *Journal of Biological Chemistry* 231:241–257, 1958.

28. Olby, *Francis Crick*, p. 265.

29. Watson, J., Essay: Letter to a Young Scientist, *MIT Technology Review*, http://www.technologyreview.com/Biotech/19173/September/October2007.

30. Marshall Nirenberg Papers, National Library of Medicine, Lab Administration—General Files, Isotope Records, 1979–1984, Box 21, Folder 49, July 1957–February 1958, p. 179.

31. Yanofsky, C. and Crawford, I.P., The Effects of Deletions, Point Mutations, Reversions and Suppressor Mutations on the Two Components of the Tryptophan Synthetase of Escherichia coli, *Proceedings of the National Academy of Sciences of the United States of America* 45:1016–1026, 1959.

32. Cohen, G.N. and Monod, J., Bacterial Permeases, *Bacteriological Reviews* 21:169–194, 1957.

33. Marshall Nirenberg Papers, National Library of Medicine, Box 22, D7, VIIA, September 1959–May 1960, September 16, 1959.

34. Crick, F.H.C., Barnett, L., Brenner, S., and Watts-Tobin, R.J., General Nature of the Genetic Code for Proteins, *Nature* 192:1227–1232, 1961.

35. Lerman, L.S., Structural Considerations in the Interaction of DNA and Acridines, *Journal of Molecular Biology* 3:18–30, 1961.

36. Brenner, S., Barnett, L., Crick, F.H.C., and Orgel, A., The Theory of Mutagenesis, *Journal of Molecular Biology* 3:121–124, 1961.

37. Olby, *Francis Crick*, p. 284.

38. Ibid, p. 296–297.

Chapter 6

1. Harris, R., Marshall Nirenberg Interview, National Library of Medicine, 1995–1996.

2. Marshall Nirenberg Papers, National Library of Medicine, Box 21, MS C 566, D4, IV, A Series, July 1957–February 1958, index pages.

3. Ibid, p. 37.

4. Ibid, p. 66.

5. Ibid, p. 82.

6. Ibid, p. 106.

7. Ibid, p. 146.

8. Ibid, p. 179.

9. Marshall Nirenberg Papers, National Library of Medicine, Lab Research, D5, VA, October 1957–November 21, 1958, Folder 50, index pages.

10. Ibid, p. 12.

11. Ibid, p. 35.

12. Ibid, pp. 121–122.

13. Ibid, p. 144.

14. Jakoby, W., interview with author, June 12, 2012.

15. Marshall Nirenberg Papers, National Library of Medicine, Lab Research, D5, VA, October 1957–November 21, 1958, Folder 50, p. 161.

16. Ibid, p. 169.

17. Ibid, p. 189.

18. Calvin, M., personal communication, 1966.

19. Marshall Nirenberg Papers, National Library of Medicine, Lab Research, Lab Diaries, D6, VI A, Box 22, Folder 1, November 1958–December 1959, p. 1.

20. Ibid, p. 83.

21. Ibid, p. 84.

22. Ibid, p. 85.

23. Ibid, p. 100.

Chapter 7

1. Hastings, J.W., William David McElroy, January 22, 1917–February 17, 1999, National Academy of Sciences, Biographical Memoirs., vol. 85, pp. 172–173.

2. Portugal, F., Oswald T. Avery: Nobel Laureate or Noble Luminary?, *Perspectives in Biology and Medicine*, 53:558–570, 2010.

3. McElroy, W.D. and Glass, B., *A Symposium on the Chemical Basis of Heredity*, The Johns Hopkins Press, Baltimore, 1957, pp. 200–231.

4. Ibid, pp. 232–267.

5. Ibid, pp. 268–275.

6. Ibid, pp. 232–267.

7. Ibid, pp. 501–512.

8. Ibid, p. 527.

9. Ibid, p. 528.

10. Ibid, pp. 615–638.

11. Ibid, pp. 686–695.

12. Harris, R., Marshall Nirenberg Interview, National Library of Medicine, 1995–1996.

13. Dryer, W., interview, http://resolver.caltech.edu/CaltechOH:OH_Dreyer_W.

14. Ames, B., interview with author, December 29, 2011.

15. Marshall Nirenberg Papers, National Library of Medicine, Box 22, D7, VIIA, September 1959–May 1960, October 22, 1959, p. 20.

16. Sanger, F. and Thompson, E.O., The Amino-Acid Sequence in the Glycyl Chain of Insulin. I. The Identification of Lower Peptides from Partial Hydrolysates, *Biochemical Journal* 53:353–366, 1953.

17. Lamborg, M.R. and Zamecnik, P.C., Amino Acid Incorporation into Protein by Extracts of E. coli, *Biochimica et Biophysica Acta* 42:206–211, 1960.

18. Marshall Nirenberg Papers, National Library of Medicine, Box 22, D8, VIII8A, April—September 1960, pp. 137 and 187.

19. Weissbach, A., A Novel System for the Incorporation of Amino Acids by Extracts of E. coli B, *Biochimica et Biophysica Acta* 41:498–509, 1960.

20. Marshall Nirenberg Papers, National Library of Medicine, Box 22, D8, VIIIA, April—September 1960, August 8, 1960, p. 128.

21. Marshall Nirenberg Papers, National Library of Medicine, Box 22, D9, IXA, September 1960–May 1961, p. 19.

22. Ibid, p. 31.

23. Marshall Nirenberg Papers, National Library of Medicine, Box 22, D8, VIIA, September 1959–May 1960, September 24, 1959.

24. Ibid, p. 6.

25. Ibid, October 22, 1959, p. 22.

26. Ibid, p. 37.

27. Ibid, p. 125.

28. Ibid, p. 160.

29. Ibid, March 26, 1960, p. 184.

30. Ibid, p. 85.

31. Hoagland, M.B., Stephenson, M.L., Scott, J.F., and Zamernik, P.C., A Soluble Ribonucleic Acid Intermediate in Protein Synthesis, *Journal of Biological Chemistry* 231:241–257, 1958.

32. Jacob, F., Perrin, D., Sanchez, C, and Monod, J., Operon: A Group of Genes with the Expression Coordinated by an Operator, *Comptes rendus hebdomadaires des séances de l'Académie des sciences* 250:1727–1729, 1960.

33. McQuillen, K, Roberts, R.B., and Britten, R.J., Synthesis of Nascent Protein by Ribosomes in Escherichia coli, *Proceedings of the National Academy of Sciences of the United States of America* 45:1437–1447, 1959.

34. Deciphering the Genetic Code: In the Late Marshall Nirenberg's Own Words, *The NIH Catalyst,* March–April 2010, pp. 6–7.

35. Marshall Nirenberg Papers, National Library of Medicine, Box 22, D8, VIIIA, April–September 1960, p. 36.

36. Ibid, May 23, 1960, p. 27.

37. Ibid, May 26, 1960, p. 34.

38. Ibid, p. 90.

39. Ibid, p. 95.

40. Ibid, p 121.

41. Ibid, p. 126.

42. Ibid, p. 128.

43. Ibid, p. 145.

44. Marshall Nirenberg Papers, National Library of Medicine, Lab Administration—General Files, Isotope Records, 1979–1984, Box 21, Folder 49, July 1957–February 1958, p. 189.

45. Marshall Nirenberg papers, National Library of Medicine, Box 22, D9, IXA, September 1960–May 1961, November 4, 1960 (referencing November 5), p. 15.

46. Ibid, p. 14.

47. Ibid, p. 20.

48. Ibid, p. 21.

49. Matthaei, H., personal communication, October 29, 2013.

50. Marshall Nirenberg Papers, National Library of Medicine, Box 22, D8, VIIIA, April–September 1960, p. 114.

51. F.H. Crick to Arthur Kornberg, May 10, 1960, Profiles in Science, The National Library of Medicine, http://profiles.nlm.nih.gov/ps/access/SCBBGZ.pdf.

52. Marshall Nirenberg Papers, National Library of Medicine, Box 22, D8, VIIIA, April—September 1960, p. 27.

53. Friedberg, E.C., Research Highlights: An Interview with Marshall Nirenberg, *Nature Reviews Molecular Cell Biology*, 9:190, 2008.

54. Matthaei, H. and Nirenberg, M.W., The Dependence of Cell-Free Protein Synthesis in *E. coli* upon RNA Prepared from Ribosomes, *Biochemical and Biophysical Research Communications* 4:404–408, 1961.

55. Fritz Lipmann to F.H.C. Crick, November 27, 1961, Profiles in Science, The National Library of Medicine, http://profiles.nlm.nih.gov/ps/retrieve/Resource Metadata/SCBBBV#transcript.

56. Matthaei and Nirenberg, M., Dependence of Cell-Free Protein Synthesis, p. 406.

57. Gros, F, Hiatt, H., Gilbert, W., Kurkland, C.G., Risebrough, R.W., and Watson J.D., Unstable Ribonucleic Acid Revealed by Pulse Labeling of *Escherichia coli*, *Nature* 190:581–585, 1961.

58. Brenner, S., Jacob, F. and Meselson, M., An Unstable Intermediate Carrying Information from Genes to Ribosomes for Protein Synthesis, *Nature* 190:576–581, 1961.

59. Marshall Nirenberg Papers, National Library of Medicine, D8, VIIIA, April–September 1960, p. 146.

60. Ibid, p. 153.

61. Marshall Nirenberg Papers, National Library of Medicine, MWN Papers, Box 22, D9, IXA, September 1960–May 1961, p. 46.

62. Felsenfeld, G., personal communication, December 5, 2013.

63. Matthaei, J.H. and Nirenberg, M.W., Characteristics and Stabilization of DNA-ase-sensitive Protein Synthesis in E. coli extracts. *Proceedings of the National Academy of Sciences of the United States of America* 47:1580–1588, 1961.

64. Marshall Nirenberg Papers, National Library of Medicine, Box 22, D9, IXA, September 1960–May 1961, January 13, 1961, Box 22, p. 89.

65. Matthaei, H., personal communication, February 28, 2010.

66. Nirenberg, M.W. and Matthaei, J.H., The Dependence of Cell-Free Protein Synthesis in E. coli upon Naturally Occurring or Synthetic Polyribonucleotides, *Proceedings of the National Academy of Sciences of the United States of America*, 47:1588–1602, 1961.

67. Crick, F.H.C., Barnett, L., Brenner, S., and Watts-Tobin, R.J., General Nature of the Genetic Code for Proteins, *Nature* 192:1227–1232, 1961.

68. Matthaei, H., personal communication, May 18, 2012.

69. Ibid., March 3, 2010.

70. Ibid., June 16, 2012.

71. Matthaei, H., personal communication, October 29, 2013.

Chapter 8

1. Deciphering the Genetic Code: In the Late Marshall Nirenberg's Own Words, *The NIH Catalyst*, March–April 2010, pp. 6–7.

2. Agranoff, B., Draft of article for UM Department of Biological Chemistry 2010 Newsletter, personal communication, February 24, 2010.

3. Fifth International Congress of Biochemistry, vol. 9, Plenary Sessions and Abstracts of Papers, Pergamon Press, Oxford, 1963, p. 7.

4. Ibid, p. 102.

5. Meselson, M., interview with author, January 29, 2013.

6. Harris, R., Marshall Nirenberg Interview, National Library of Medicine, 1995–1996.

7. Trupin, J., interview with author, October 21, 2011.

8. Greenhouse, L., interview with author, November 21, 2011.

9. Marshall Nirenberg Papers, National Library of Medicine, Box 22, D11 XA, June–December 1961, September 16, 1961, pp. 58–61.

10. Grunberg-Manago, Marianne; Ortiz, P, Ochoa, S., Enzymic Synthesis of Polynucleotides. I. Polynucleotide Phosphorylase of Azotobacter vinelandii, *Biochemica et Biophysica Acta* 20: 269–285, 1956.

11. Grunberg-Manago, M.; Oritz, P. J.; Ochoa, S., Enzymatic Synthesis of Nucleic Acid-like Polynucleotides. *Science* 122 (3176): 907–910, 1955.

12. Emily Langer, Neuroscientist Discovered the First Brain Receptor, Obituary, *Washington Post*, September 19, 2013, page H7.

13. Beljanski, M. and Ochoa, S., Protein Biosynthesis by a Cell-Free Bacterial System, *Proceedings of the National Academy of Sciences of the United States of America* 44:494–501, 1958.

14. Lengyel, P., Memories of a Senior Scientist: On Passing the Fiftieth Anniversary of the Beginning of Deciphering the Genetic Code, *Annual Reviews of Microbiology* 66:27–38, 2012.

15. Ibid, p. 15.

16. Matthaei, J.H., Jones, O.W., Marin, R.G., and Nirenberg, M., Characteristics and Composition of RNA Coding Units, *Proceedings of the National Academy of Sciences of the United States of America* 48:666–672, 1962.

17. Marshall Nirenberg Papers, Box 22, D11, XA, June–December 1961, September 16, 1961, p. 88.

18. Feng, A.S., The ISN President's Column, *International Society for Neuroethology*, November 2002, p. 5.

19. Nirenberg, M., Historical Review: Deciphering the Genetic Code—A Personal Account, *Trends in Biochemical Sciences* 29:46–54, 2004, p. 49.

20. Lengyel, P., Speyer, J.F., and Ochoa, S., Synthetic Polynucleotides and the Amino Acid Code, *Proceedings of the National Academy of Sciences of the United States of America* 47:1936–1942, 1961.

21. Marshall Nirenberg Papers, National Library of Medicine, Box 22, D11, XA, June–December 1961, September 16, 1961, p. 86.

22. Ibid, p. 88.

23. Lengyel, Speyer, J.F., Memories of a Senior Scientist, p. 32.

24. Speyer, J.F., Lengyel, P., Basilio, C., and Ochoa, S., Synthetic Polynucleotides and the Amino Acid Code, II, *Proceedings of the National Academy of Sciences of the United States of America* 48:441–498, 1962.

25. Ochoa, S., The Chemical Basis of Heredity—The Genetic Code, *Bulletin of the New York Academy of Medicine* 40:387–411, 1964.

Chapter 9

1. Olby, R., *Francis Crick: Hunter of Life's Secrets*, Cold Spring Harbor Laboratory Press, New York, 2009, p. 285.

2. Klein, M.K., The Legacy of the "Yellow Berets," manuscript 1998, NIH History Office, National Institutes of Maryland, Bethesda, Maryland.

3. Levin, J., interview with author, February 6, 2013.

4. Ames, B., interview with author, December 29, 2011.

5. Martin, R., interview with author, November 22, 2011.

6. Martin, R.G., A Revisionist View of the Breaking of the Genetic Code, in *NIH: An Account of Research in Its Laboratories and Clinics*, eds. DeWitt Stetten, Jr. and W.T. Carrigan, Academic Press, 1984, p. 281.

7. Harris, R., Marshall Nirenberg Interview, National Library of Medicine, 1995–1996.

8. Davies, D.R., interview with author, February 2, 2012.

9. Jones, O.W. and Nirenberg, M.W., Qualitative Survey of RNA Code Words, *Proceedings of the National Academy of Sciences of the United States of America* 48:2115–2123, 1962.

10. Marshall Nirenberg Papers, National Library of Medicine, D12, 7A, December 1961–May 1962, pp. 137–138.

11. Jones, O.W., interview with author, October 31, 2011.

12. Marshall Nirenberg Papers, National Library of Medicine, Box 22, D13, 8A, May–September 1962, p. 10.

13. Ibid, p.11.

14. Ibid, pp. 11–13.

15. Ibid, p. 54.

16. Roberts, R.B., Alternative Codes and Templates, *Proceedings of the National Academy of Sciences of the United States of America* 48:897–900, 1962.

17. Torgan, C., 1960's Lab Life with the Nobel Prize-Winning Decipherer of the Genetic Code. Guest post by Norma Zabriskie Heaton, http://www.caroltorgan.com/genetic-code-decipherer-lab-life.

18. Marshall Nirenberg Papers, National Library of Medicine, Box 22, D13, 8A, May–September 1962, p. 30.

19. Gallo, R., interview with author, May 26, 2011.

20. Marshall Nirenberg Papers, National Library of Medicine, Box 22, D11, XA, June–December 1961, p. 58.

21. Ibid, 61.

22. Ibid, p. 79.

23. Ibid, p. 85.

24. Ibid, 86–87.

25. Crick, F.H.C., On the Genetic Code, *Nobel Lectures, Physiology or Medicine 1942–1962*, Elsevier Publishing Company, Amsterdam, 1964.

26. Marshall Nirenberg Papers, National Library of Medicine, Box 22, D11, XA, June–December 1961, p. 131.

27. Ibid, p. 158.

28. O'Neal, C., interview with author, January 26, 2012.

29. Felsenfeld, G., interview with author, November 20, 2012.

30. Marshall Nirenberg Papers, National Library of Medicine, Box 22, D12, 7A, December 1961–May 1962, p. 157.

31. Marshall Nirenberg Papers, National Library of Medicine, Box 22, D13, 8A, May–September 1962, p. 44.

32. Clark, B., interview with author, October 9, 2011.

33. Marshall Nirenberg Papers, National Library of Medicine, Box 22, D12, 7A, December 1961–May 1962, p. 93.

34. Ibid, p. 35.

35. Ibid, p. 134.

36. Weissbach, H. and Witkop, B., Sidney Udenfriend, *Biographical Memoirs*, vol. 83:1–29, 2003, National Academies Press, Washington, D.C. 2003, pg. 271–298.

37. Marshall Nirenberg Papers, National Library of Medicine, Maurice Niehuss to Marshall Nirenberg, May 19, 1961.

38. 1/15/10 Marshall Nirenberg, 1968 Nobel Laureate, Dies, http://www .improbablebooks.com/newsserotonin.html.

39. Marshall Nirenberg Papers, National Library of Medicine, Box 22, D15, 9A September 1962–January 1963, p.11.

40. Ibid, p. 12.

41. Ibid, p. 18.

42. Ibid, p. 27.

43. Marshall Nirenberg Papers, National Library of Medicine, Box 22, D12, 7A, December 1961–May 1962, p. 135.

44. Leder, P., interview with author, May 16, 2012.

45. Leder, P., Marshall Warren Nirenberg (1927–2010), *Science* 327:972, 2010.

46. Marshall Nirenberg Papers, National Library of Medicine, Box 22, D13, 8A, May–September 1962, p. 55.

47. Ibid, p. 127.

48. Ibid, p. 161.

49. Ibid, p. 156.

50. Marshall Nirenberg Papers, National Library of Medicine, Box 22, D15, 9A September 1962–January 1963, p. 27.

51. Marshall Nirenberg Papers, National Library of Medicine, Box 22, D17, 11A, April–June 1963, p. 151.

52. Marshall Nirenberg Papers, National Library of Medicine, Box 22, D18, 12A, July–November 1963, p. 131.

53. Marshall Nirenberg Papers, National Library of Medicine, Box 22, D20, 13A, Index, November 1963–April 1964, p. 16.

54. Marshall Nirenberg Papers, National Library of Medicine, Box 22, Folder 15, D20, 13A, Lab Research-Lab Diaries, November 1963–April 1964, p. 3.

55. Ibid., p. 39.

56. Portugal, F.H. and Cohen, J.S., *A Century of DNA*, MIT Press, 1977, pp. 298–299.

57. Trupin, J., interview with author, October 21, 2011.

58. Marshall Nirenberg Papers, National Library of Medicine, Box 22, D21, 14A, April–October 1964, Folder 16, Lab Research-Lab Diaries, Index, pp. 1–8.

59. Ibid., p. 13.

60. Ibid., p. 152.

61. Marshall Nirenberg Papers, National Library of Medicine, Box 22, Folder 15, D20, 13A, Lab Research-Lab Diaries, November 1963–April 1964, p. 41.

62. Ibid, p. 176.

63. Ibid, p. 67.

64. Ibid, p. 72.

65. Ibid, p. 43.

66. Ibid, p. 51.

67. Scolnick, E., interview with author, December 11, 2012.

68. Marshall Nirenberg Papers, National Library of Medicine, Box 23, Folder 1, D22, 15A, Lab Research-Lab Diaries, October 9 1964 –January 9 1965, Index, p. 13.

69. Ibid, p. 31.

70. Crick, F.H.C., On the Genetic Code, *Science* 139:461–464, 1963.

71. Olby, *Francis Crick*, p. 301.

72. Crick, F.H., Codon-Anticodon Pairing: The Wobble Hypothesis, *Journal of Molecular Biology* 19:548–555, 1966.

73. Olby, *Francis Crick*, p. 297.

74. Ridley, M., *Francis Crick: Discoverer of the Genetic Code*, Harper-Collins, New York, 2006, p. 138.

75. Ibid, pp. 138–139.

76. Marshall Nirenberg Papers, National Library of Medicine, Box 23, Folder 1, D22, 15A, Lab Research-Lab Diaries, October 9, 1964 –January 9, 1965, p. 80.

77. Marshall W. Nirenberg 1968–Seattle, http://www.waymarking.com/waymarks/ WMC1F3_Physiology_Medicine_Marshall_W_Nirenberg_1968_Seattle_WA.

78. Nirenberg, M.W., Matthaei, J.H., and Jones, O.W., An Intermediate in the Biosynthesis of Polyphenylalanine Directed by Synthetic Template RNA, *Proceedings of the National Academy of Sciences of the United States of America* 48:104–109, 1962.

79. Caskey, T., interview with author, October 31, 2012.

80. Marshall, R.E., Caskey, C.T., and Nirenberg, M., Fine Structure of RNA Codewords Recognized by Bacterial, Amphibian, and Mammalian Transfer RNA, *Science* 155:820–826, 1967.

81. Caskey, T., Scolnick, E., Tompkins, R., Goldstein, J., and Milman, G., Peptide Chain Termination: Codon, Protein Factor, and Ribosomal Requirements, *Cold Spring Harbor Symposium on Quantitative Biology* 34:479–488, 1969.

82. Beaudet, A., interview with author, January 14, 2013.

83. Goldstein, J., interview with author, November 7, 2012.

84. Goldstein, J. and Brown, M., A Golden Era of Nobel Laureates, *Science* 338:1033–1034, 2012.

Chapter 10

1. Marshall Nirenberg Papers, National Library of Medicine, Box 22, D7, VIIA, September 1959–May 1960, p. 7.

2. Marshall Nirenberg Papers, National Library of Medicine, Box 22, D15, 9A, September 1962–January 1963, p. 103.

3. Marshall Nirenberg Papers, National Library of Medicine, Box 22, D18, 12A, July–November 1963, p. 21.

4. Ibid, p. 99.

5. Marshall Nirenberg Papers, National Library of Medicine, Box 22, Folder 14, Lab Research-Lab Diaries, D19, I, Brain, 12A-2, Sept. 20–28, 1963, Index, p. 1.

6. Ibid, p. 3.

7. Torgan, C., 1960s Lab Life with the Nobel Prize-Winning Decipherer of the Genetic Code. Guest post by Norma Zabriskie Heaton, http://www.caroltorgan.com/genetic-code-decipherer-lab-life.

8. Augusti-Tocco, G. and Sato, G., Establishment of Functional Clonal Lines of Neurons from Mouse Neuroblastoma, *Proceedings of the National Academy of Sciences of the United States of America.*, 64:311–315, 1969.

9. Nelson, P., Ruffner, W., and Nirenberg, M., Neuronal Tumor Cells with Excitable Membranes Grown in Vitro, *Proceedings of the National Academy of Sciences of the United States of America* 64: 1004–1010, 1969.

10. Minna, J., Nelson, P., Peacock, J., Glazer, D., and Nirenberg, M., Genes for Neronal Properties Expressed in Neuroblastoma x L Cell Hybrids, *Proceedings of the National Academy of Sciences of the United States of America* 68:234–239, 1971.

11. Nelson, P., Christian, C, and Nirenberg, M., Synapse Formation Between Clonal Neuroblastoma x Glioma Cells and Striated Muscle, *Proceedings of the National Academy of Sciences of the United States of America* 73:123–127, 1976.

12. Nelson, P., interview with author, January 23, 2013.

13. Moskal, J.R., Trisler, D., Schneider, M.D., and Nirenberg, M., Purification of a Membrane Protein Distributed in a Topographic Gradient in Chicken Retina, *Proceedings of the National Academy of Sciences of the United States of America* 83:4730–4733, 1986.

14. Tan, D-P., Ferrante, J., Nazarali, A., Shao, X., Kozak, C.A., Guo, V., and Nirenberg, M., Murine *Hox-1.11* Homeobox Gene Structure and Expression, *Proceedings of the National Academy of Sciences of the United States of America* 89:6280–6284, 1992.

15. Rovescalli, A.C., Asoh, S., and Nirenberg, M., Cloning and Characterization of Four Murine Homeobox Genes, *Proceedings of the National Academy of Sciences of the United States of America* 93:10691–10696, 1996.

16. Lum, L., Yao, S., Mozer, B., Rovescalli, A., Von Kessler, D., Nirenberg, M., and Beachy, P.A., Identification of Hedgehog Pathway Components by RNAi in Drosophila Cultured Cells, *Science* 299:2039–2045, 2003.

17. Ivanov, A.I. Rovescalli, A.C., Pozzi, P., Yoo, S., Mozer, B., Li, H-P., Yu, S-H., Higashida, H., Guo, V., Spencer, M., and Nirenberg, M., Genes Required for Drosophila Nervous System Development Identified by RNA Interference, *Proceedings of the National Academy of Sciences of the United States of America* 101:16216–16221, 2004.

18. Weiss, R., Nobel Laureates Back Stem Cell Research; Group of 80 Recipients Sends Letter Asking Bush Not to Block U.S. Funding for Studies, *Washington Post*, February 22, 2001, p. A02.

19. Weissman, M., interview with author, August 19 and 22, 2013.

20. Koizumi, K., Higashida, H., Yoo, S., Islam, M.S., Ivanov, A.I., Guo, V., Pozzi, P., Yu, S-H., Rovescalli, A.C., Tang, D., and Nirenberg, M., RNA Interference Screen to Identify Genes Required for *Drosophila Melanogaster* Embryonic Nervous System Development, *Proceedings of the National Academy of Sciences of the United States of America* 104:5626–5631, 2007.

21. Xia, M., Huang, R., Guo, V., Southall, N., Cho, M-H., Inglese, J., Austin, C.P., and Nirenberg, M., Identification of Compounds that Potentiate CREB Signaling as Possible Enhancers of Long-Term Memory, *Proceedings of the National Academy of Sciences of the United States of America* 106:2412–2417, 2009.

22. Xia, M., Guo, V., Huang, R., Shahane, S.A., Austin, C.P., Nirenberg, M., and Sharma, S.K., Inhibition of Morphine-induced cAMP Overshoot: A Cell-based Assay Model in a High-Throughput Format, *Cellular and Molecular Neurobiology* 31:901–907, 2011.

23. Olby, R., *Francis Crick: Hunter of Life's Secrets*, Cold Spring Harbor Laboratory Press, New York, 2009, p. 377.

24. Ibid, p. 383.

25. Ibid, p. 359–360.

26. Ibid, p. 369.

27. Crick, F. and Mitchison, G., The Function of Dream Sleep, *Nature* 301:111–114, 1983.

28. Crick, F., Function of the Thalamic Reticular Complex: The Searchlight Hypothesis, *Proceedings of the National Academy of Sciences of the United States of America* 81:4586–4590, 1984.

29. Rafal, R.D. and Posner, M.I., Deficits in Human Visual Spatial Attention Following Thalamic Lesions (Selective Attention), *Proceedings of the National Academy of Sciences of the United States of America* 84:7349–7353, 1987.

30. Olby, *Francis Crick*, p. 407.

31. Crick, F. and Koch, C., Toward a Neurobiological Theory of Consciousness, *Seminars in Neuroscience* 2:263–275, 1990.

32. Olby, *Francis Crick*, p. 409.

33. Crick, F.C. and Koch, C., What Is the Function of the Claustrum?, *Philosophical Transactions of the Royal Society B* 360:1271–1279, 2005.

34. Koch, C., Book Review: In the Playing Ground of Consciousness, *Science* 343:487, 2014.

35. Amamoto, R. and Arlotta, P., Development-Inspired Reprogramming of the Mammalian Central Nervous System, *Science* 343:1239882, 2014.

Chapter 11

1. Cosmos Club, https://www.cosmosclub.org/Default.aspx?pageindex=1&pageid=111&status=1.

2. The Townsend Mansion, Cosmos Club, https://www.cosmosclub.org/Default.aspx?pageid=75&pageindex=0.

3. The Marshall W. Nirenberg Papers, Beyond the Laboratory: Personal, Professional, and Political Life, 1967–2002, National Library of Medicine, http://profiles.nlm.nih.gov/ps/retrieve/Narrative/JJ/p-nid/83.

4. McArdle, D., Cosmos Club: Women Members?, *Washington Post-Times Herald*, December 31, 1972, p. E6.

5. Weiser, B., Cosmos Club to Remain a Bastion for Men Only, *Washington Post*, December 18, 1980, p. B1.

6. Saperstein, S., Cosmos Club Lifts Member's Reprimand, *Washington Post,* January 23, 1986, p. C1.

7. Feinberg, L., Cosmos Club Attacked by D.C. Ruling, *Washington Post,* November 7, 1987, p. G1.

Index